SKIN DEEP

The essential guide to what's really in the toiletries and cosmetics you use

PAT THOMAS

This edition first published 2008 by Rodale
an imprint of Pan Macmillan Ltd
Pan Macmillan, 20 New Wharf Road, London N1 9RR
Basingstoke and Oxford
Associated companies throughout the world
www.panmacmillan.com

ISBN 978-1-9057-44-23-7

Portions of the text in this book were published previously in *What's In This Stuff?* by
Pat Thomas, also published by Rodale.

Chemical names that appear in italics are listed in Appendix 2, 'Chemicals A–Z'.

1 3 5 7 9 8 6 4 2

A CIP catalogue record for this book is available from the British Library.

Printed and bound in the UK by CPI Mackays, Chatham ME5 8TD

This book is intended as a reference volume only, not as a medical manual. The information
given here is designed to help you make informed decisions about your health. It is not
intended as a substitute for any treatment that you may have been prescribed by your doctor.
If you suspect you have a medical problem, we urge you to seek competent medical help.
Mention of specific companies, organizations or authorities in this book does not imply
endorsement of the publisher, nor does mention of specific companies, organizations or
authorities in the book imply that they endorse the book.
Addresses, websites and telephone numbers given in this book were correct at the time of
going to press.

Visit *www.panmacmillan.com* to read more about all our books and to buy them. You will
also find features, author interviews and news of any author events, and you can sign up for
e-newsletters so that you're always first to hear about our new releases.

We inspire and enable people to improve their lives and the world around them

Acknowledgements

Writing a book requires the support of family, friends and colleagues all of whom are prepared to tolerate various sorts of absences – physical, mental and emotional. Love and thanks to the wonderful 'constants' in my galaxy of stars, my son Alex, my agent Laura Longrigg, and my dear friends and colleagues at the *Ecologist* and to the hardest working Bull in show business. Gratitude also to Liz Gough and all at Pan Macmillan for support and a guiding hand along the way.

Other Rodale books by Pat Thomas

What's In This Stuff?
Healthy, Happy Baby

Contents

PART ONE

Introduction

We use them to make us feel good, smell good and look good. We spend vast amounts of money on them – globally more than $200 billion a year – and with that investment comes a lot of blind faith that all the toiletries and beauty products we use on our hair, our skin, indeed all over our bodies, will provide an instant make-over. Whatever our heads may know, our hearts still want to believe that there is some quick-fix magic in the products we buy that will – at least for a little while – make us younger, sexier, more beautiful (or more handsome) and more vibrant than before.

The expectation of magic in all our personal-care products is strong, and the promises on the front of the package are so seductive that most of us never bother to check out what they are actually made from. Chances are, even if you do check the label of your favourite cosmetics, all you will see is an incomprehensible, alphabet soup of unpronounceable words.

It's easier, and certainly more comforting, to believe in some vague magic than it is to learn to make sense of the often impenetrable labels on personal-care products. But the effort might just be worth making, since regardless of the package's come-on, achieving a cosmetic quick-fix requires a cocktail of largely synthetic ingredients which have been linked with longer term health concerns.

For many years I have made my living lifting the lid on the products we buy and use every day. So I feel fortunate to have a broad understanding of the cumulative effects – environmentally and in terms of human health – of a lifetime's exposure to synthetic chemicals. Looking at the science and the psychology of consumer goods and the society in which they flourish is both fascinating and worrying. I've never been able to get to grips with why we buy so much, why we use so much and why we put things on our bodies (and *in* our bodies) without ever questioning what is in them or what happens to them when they go down the drain.

The individual chemicals in personal-care products are a particularly insidious form of body pollution because they enter the body through multiple routes. We can swallow them, inhale them and absorb them through the skin as well as through the mucous membranes in the eyes, mouth and nose. The absorption of substances through the skin and mucous membranes is particularly disturbing, because the body's normal filters – the kidneys and liver – are bypassed.

In addition, the mix of chemicals in the products we use can make the problem worse. Many toiletries contain a cocktail of emollients (oils and fats), solvents (for instance *propylene glycol*) and humectants (such as *glycerine*) which, while relatively harmless in their own right, together increase the skin's permeability, and therefore increase the amount of other more toxic ingredients found in the mix which can be absorbed into the bloodstream. To help demystify these substances, see the 'Chemicals A–Z' on p. 143.

In an ideal world, we would all be able to judge the safety of a product by its labelling. Unfortunately, manufacturers are very inconsistent in their labelling practices and many actively resist full-disclosure of ingredients on the label because of the fear of a customer backlash. What this means is that on any supermarket shelf you will find some products where the labels are printed on the container, and others where they are listed on peel-away labels on the underside of the product. Others list them on the box (which often gets thrown away without a glance), some use vague wording (like 'natural extracts') or worse don't list their ingredients at all, or only make ingredient lists available on request at the point of sale (a common practice with make-up).

Similarly, while many people assume that there is a government department somewhere overseeing the safety and effectiveness of personal-care products, this is not true. The companies that produce toiletries and cosmetics are largely self-regulating. Beyond enforcing guidelines about what ingredients not to use, most regulatory agencies don't require manufacturers to prove that their products are either safe or effective.

The skeletal regulations that do exist do little to protect consumers, especially over the longer term. For instance, while regulators have approved more than 3,000 ingredients for cosmetic use in Europe, many more substances find their way into our cosmetics and toiletries through loopholes in the law – for instance those that allow products to contain traces of contaminants and other banned substances that are difficult to remove during or after manufacture.

What all this means is that it is currently very difficult for all but the most motivated among us to make good decisions about what products to buy. That's where this book comes in.

In the first section we take an in-depth look at the way products are made, taking apart the key ingredients in the beauty products we use, from preservatives to humectants, from detergents to emulsifiers. Each type of ingredient has a role to play in formulating the finished product, but as toiletries and beauty products have become more and more mass-produced, the choice of ingredient is often driven more by price than by safety or even how well it works. The good news, as you will see, is that there are many good, safe, effective natural alternatives to the

LIFTING THE LID

Your skin absorbs up to 60 per cent of the chemicals that come into contact with it and sends them directly into the bloodstream. Research suggests it can take as little as 26 seconds for some of these substances to go from the skin to every major organ of the body. Women – who use more toiletries and cosmetics than men – are thought to absorb around 2kg of cosmetic ingredients each year.

chemical ingredients we use every day. By using the information in this section you will be able to identify these on the products you buy with greater ease.

The second section tackles the products we buy and use every day. It uncovers the mixture of chemicals in products such as a typical shampoo, face cream or toothpaste, and explains how they can be even more harmful to your health and the environment when used together. You will understand the psychology of beauty-product advertising, read how to make safer choices, be encouraged to use simpler alternatives (including the alternative of not using certain products at all – for instance how much do you really need a conditioner for your hair?) and be offered quick DIY recipes for natural beauty to help you break your dependence on potentially dangerous products.

At the end of the book are invaluable resources to help you decode the labels of your favourite brands.

You may be startled by what you read, yet taking these facts on board has important implications for your health today, for the health of future generations and for the health of the planet. Learning about the ingredients in the products we buy and use every day can help you become a canny consumer. You will find that as you get to grips with what at first may appear to be complex information, your life will become infinitely less complicated.

For me, information is power. My hope is that by lifting the lid on the products you use, you will feel empowered to look differently at the products you use, to read the labels on them with confidence, to know when you really need a product and when you can opt for a more natural, less toxic life.

Good luck and good health.

Chapter 1

The Burden of Beauty

There was probably a time when all we needed to get cleaned up and ready for the day was a bit of soap and water (and in reality we still don't need much more than that!). Today, however, we use dozens of products with potentially hundreds of chemical ingredients in them. If you are a typical woman your beauty routine may involve using anything between 10 and 20 different products and you could be exposing yourself to upward of 200 potentially harmful chemicals each day.

We use these products in vast quantities every day without thinking, and because of this we are exposed to a wide variety of chemicals that were never meant to be in our bodies.

Skin is the largest organ in the body, and while we think of our skin as a barrier, in fact it can absorb a significant amount of whatever we put onto it. Modern toiletries use substances called penetration enhancers to alter the way that skin absorbs chemicals. These are added to products specifically to drive ingredients deeper into the skin and produce the quick-fix effects – for instance the promise of a decrease in visible wrinkles in one hour – that we have come to expect from modern cosmetics.

When applied, they contribute to what is called your 'body burden' or your 'total toxic load' which is the total amount of chemicals present in your body. It is impossible to say how many different man-made chemicals we each carry in our bodies. This is because beyond chemicals added to food, or those used as drugs, there is no requirement for manufacturers to disclose how their chemicals are used or keep track of the routes through which people are exposed.

Most regulatory agencies don't require manufacturers to prove that their products are either safe or effective

Studies of blood samples from average people all over the world, however, show that most of us are carrying a heavy burden of chemicals in our bodies. In the largest study of chemical exposure ever conducted on human beings, most American children and adults were carrying in their bodies more than 100 substances that aren't supposed to be there, including pesticides and the toxic compounds used in everyday consumer products. Many of these have been linked to health threats such as cancer, central nervous system disruption, birth defects and immune system damage.

These chemicals come from household products like detergents, perfumes, toiletries and cosmetics as well as fabric treatments and paints, upholstery, computers and TVs. They are 'persistent' – that is instead of breaking down, they remain intact in your body for long periods of time where they accumulate in fat, blood and organs, or are passed through the body in breastmilk, urine, faeces, sweat, semen, hair and nails. Over time, if the total body load is high, the likelihood of the body breaking down under the weight of it becomes higher.

But chemicals don't have to be present in high quantities to cause problems. Scientists have recently discovered what they call the 'low-dose effect', which suggests that even small doses of certain chemicals

LIFTING THE LID

According to government reports in both the US and EU around 90 per cent of the ingredients used in conventional cosmetics do not have a full set of long-term human safety data.

can have big repercussions on health in both the short and long term. This phenomenon has been particularly well researched in the field of hormone disruption where even minute quantities of different oestrogen mimics can produce an effect on the body that is many times greater than would be expected.

Environmental costs

While you are thinking about the human health implications of some of the products you use, don't forget the health of the planet. In recent years beauty has become an important green issue with more and more companies vying for the custom of women (and, increasingly men) who want to make natural and ethical choices in their personal-care products. Everything we use, everything we flush down the drain – and not just the ingredients in the products but the packaging they come in – has a carbon footprint. The vast majority of the products we use are derived from petrochemicals, and every manufactured product, and its packaging, requires energy to produce and ship around the world.

Detergents and surfactants, which clean and allow easier spreading over the body, are used in everything from shampoo to body lotion and are a good example. Compared to the manufacture of petrochemical-based surfactants, those derived from vegetable oils such as palm and coconut produce 17 and 23 per cent less solid waste respectively. Both palm- and coconut-derived surfactants require around 13 per cent less energy to produce.

Other evidence shows that the manufacture of soaps derived from tallow (i.e. *sodium tallowate*, an animal-fat based detergent) is responsible for substantially more emissions of CO_2 and other climate-changing gases than soaps made from vegetable-derived detergents.

It has been calculated that if the beauty industry increased its use of vegetable-based surfactants by one quarter it could cut its overall CO_2 emissions by around 8 per cent. But, because surfactants based on petrochemicals are cheaper to produce, it won't make the switch until customers make the demand.

Of course, as natural resources run out, many of our everyday choices become more complicated. For instance, to meet increasing global demand for palm oil, vast tracts of rainforest are being cut down. The cultivation of palm oil plantations for palm-derived ingredients in food and cosmetics, as well as those used in industrial applications like biofuels, causes deforestation and the destruction of vital peatlands, which act like sponges soaking up global CO_2 emissions. Deforestation and the peat fires used to clear land for palm oil plantation are responsible for around 30 per cent of global CO_2 emissions.

There are also other cosmetic ingredients that are destructive to the planet including talc, mica and aluminium – mined ingredients that increase the release of CO_2 from the soil when mined and emit climate-changing gases as they are refined. For example, making 1 tonne of aluminium (found in deodorants, glitter and cosmetics' dyes) releases 1.5 tonnes of CO_2 into the atmosphere.

Making 1 tonne of aluminium for deodorants and cosmetics' dyes releases 1.5 tonnes of CO_2 into the atmosphere

A lot of exotic cosmetic ingredients are shipped rather than flown around the world, something the cosmetics industry believes it can count on the plus side of its eco-accounting. But ships release nitrogen and sulphur – both potent climate-changing gases. By 2010 it is estimated that 40 per cent of air pollution over land could come from shipping. The more we demand exotic ingredients in our products the bigger this problem will get.

How cosmetics are made
The people who create our personal-care products are specially trained chemists called formulators. The formulator's brief is simple. Each new product needs to fulfil a specific function like make hair shine, stop body odour or whiten teeth. How that is achieved has less to do with the potential long-term impacts of the mixture and more to do with delivering a cost-effective product with a good profit margin.

When a formulator makes a new product he or she follows a recipe just like a chef creating a new dish. And as it is with food, so it is with toiletries and cosmetics – the better the quality of ingredients, the better the finished product. Unfortunately, the majority of personal-care products on the market are the beauty equivalent of junk food, made to fill a temporary craving and comprised of cheap ingredients that aren't very good for you.

LIFTING THE LID

UK consumers spend £5 billion a year on cosmetics. Yet in 2004 when the insurance company Prudential released a report that looked at waste in all aspects of our lives, an interesting fact emerged: 42 per cent of the women surveyed had bought toiletries they have never used or only used a couple of times; 18 per cent of men had done the same thing. These unused toiletries get thrown away or poured down the drain. The fossil fuel energy used to produce them has been totally wasted and the ingredients in them join the waste stream and enter our waterways as some of the most ubiquitous and harmful pollutants in our environment. The moral? Keep your personal-hygiene routine simple. It's better for you and better for the planet.

While the bright and bulging shelves of products in our supermarkets and chemists would suggest that there are thousands of different recipes, the truth is that most of these products are made from the same basic list of ingredients. In the end, there are only so many ways to make a shampoo or a toothpaste and the differences between products are often down to how manufacturers choose to advertise them, rather than what is actually in them.

Because cosmetics are largely made from industrial chemicals – substances that were never meant to come into regular contact with the human body – they have the potential to cause both short- and longer-term health problems. Certain types of ingredients, for instance, such as preservatives, perfumes and colours are known to be a significant cause of skin reactions. In fact, skin reactions are the most frequently reported adverse effect of using cosmetics and toiletries.

Furthermore, evidence suggests that the number of people experiencing skin reactions to cosmetics is increasing. Currently more than 80 per cent of those who develop reactions to cosmetics are healthy individuals without any prior skin problems.

It can be fairly easy to pinpoint the cosmetic causes of skin reactions such as dermatitis (inflammation of the skin). Tracking the causes of more significant or longer-term problems such as depression, migraines and even cancer is a much more difficult task. Yet as research into cosmetic ingredients advances, scientists are finding that many of the same substances that can cause short-term problems are poisonous in the long term. Skin reactions, then, could be seen as the body's early-warning system kicking in and telling you to stop using particular products or to avoid certain ingredients.

For all these reasons it's good to have some knowledge of what actually goes in to the products you buy and use.

A way forward

From a health perspective, as well as from an environmental perspective, the best choice is to buy less, and be very choosy about what you do buy. The simpler your personal-care routine is, the better it is likely to be for you and for the planet. Using natural products requires a certain degree of consciousness and a commitment to doing things differently and this book is full of eye-opening information and advice about how to choose safe, effective, natural products. As a general rule, if you want to lower your carbon footprint in the bathroom, as well as improve your long-term prospects for good health, then it's worth bearing the following principles in mind:

1. **Beauty begins with what goes in your body, not on it**
    Nothing you put on your skin will be as effective as what you put into it. Eating a healthy, balanced diet, getting sufficient sleep, not drinking alcohol to excess and not smoking will all make a greater contribution to your daily wellbeing and beauty than any products you apply to the surface – conventional or organic.

2. **Cut down on the number of products you use each day**
    By buying less you are exposing yourself to fewer man-made chemicals. You're also reducing demand on manufacturing and sending a powerful message to beauty companies about what you want from your products. Fewer products means less energy used in production and less waste at the end of the lifecycle. While you are at it, remember that most of us could be more frugal with the amount

of product we use. Shampoo is one good example; try using half the amount you normally use and you will still get your hair clean.

3. **Buy ethically**
   Learn to recognise manufacturers that genuinely strive to produce natural organic goods that do not exploit the planet or the people who help produce them. Vow only to spend your money on these products. Many organic products are available online and you can easily sign up to receive news about new products. Don't forget to spread the word among your friends to get them interested in this kind of shopping too.

4. **Resist the temptation of the impulse buy**
   Think before you buy. With so many products on the market it is so easy to just pop one or two into your shopping basket. Always ask yourself – do I really need another lipstick/body lotion/hair product? Most of us have bathrooms full of half-used products that we should use up first before we try new ones.

5. **Go fragrance-free**
   Fragrance chemicals are derived from petroleum, are known neurotoxins and carcinogens and are a major trigger of asthma. Removing them from your beauty routine is one of the healthiest things you can do.

6. **Make your own**
   Many basic toiletries can be made simply and easily at home with clean, natural organic ingredients. Facial and body moisturisers, bath treats, toners and masks made to your own specifications save money, air and road miles and ensure that you are not putting anything on your body that is harmful. The second part of this book has plenty of ideas to get you started.

7. **Keep out of reach of children**
   Don't start your children on the cosmetic habit too early. Children's bodies change and grow at an alarming rate. Play make-up, toiletries for tweenies, deodorants and colognes for teenage boys,

all contain an alarming number of potentially toxic chemicals. Be firm and do your best to protect your children from these products that poison the body and the mind.

8. Simplify your make-up routine

You don't need to be fully made-up every day of every week. There is no such thing as natural make-up and because of the chemicals involved it is probably a much healthier and greener choice to save make-up for special occasions. Learn to recognise and like your face without all the enhancements. If you must wear make-up, keep it simple – a sweep of mascara and a bit of lipgloss is enough to brighten up the faces of most women (see also Chapter 6).

9. Men beware

The male grooming market is becoming almost as crowded with products as the women's market. Apart from the packaging and the 'sell' there is no real difference between 'men's products' and 'women's products'. They contain all the same types of ingredients, including the potential carcinogens and oestrogen mimics that have been shown to 'feminise' male animals and amphibians in scientific and medical studies.

10. Don't expect natural products to work in the same way

Natural, organic products don't promise the quick-fix element that conventional ones often do and you may have to experiment to find the brands that perform the way you want them to. They can't and don't promise visible results in an hour, a day or a week. Instead, they work by supporting and maintaining the skin and hair in a healthy state. Because they don't use synthetic chemicals like silicones they may not feel the same on your skin either and you will, at first, need to learn to use them differently to get the best out of them.

11. Resist the hype

The advertising of beauty products is intended to make you feel ugly. Studies in the US have found that 70 per cent of women surveyed felt worse about their looks after reading women's magazines. That is because the emphasis is always on achieving some airbrushed, unachievable perfection. When you see a new product that promises to make you look 20 years younger, allow yourself to be a little cynical. Women in particular have a huge but not impossible job of learning to love our natural state and to celebrate variety and individuality rather than conformity. Nature loves variety; only the beauty industry loves conformity.

12. Make a list

You can use this book to identify ingredients you would prefer to avoid. Keep this list in your head or in your handbag for whenever you go shopping. Simply vowing to avoid these makes the list of things you 'need' much simpler!

Some of the information that follows may seem startling to you. But the purpose of this book is to help you think differently – and hopefully more critically – about the products that you use each day for yourself and for your family. The first part of this book lifts the lid on how products are made by exploring the broad types of ingredients that go into making personal-care products – things like preservatives, colours and fragrances. It doesn't matter whether the product is for a man, woman or child, all personal-care products contain the same types of ingredients, and these chapters offer insight into the potential health effects of some of these ingredients and lists natural alternatives that are safer.

Remember that the emphasis is on your total toxic load. It's not just single products that are the problem, but the cumulative effects of all the products we use on a daily basis that is important.

The second half of the book provides a more in-depth look at the products themselves, offering suggestions for cutting down or cutting them out altogether. Here you will find advice on doing everything from brushing your teeth to washing your hair in a less chemically intensive way. You will also find tips and recipes for making simple alternatives as well as a wealth of resources that could help you change your health and beauty routine forever, and for the better.

GOOD FOODS FOR GREAT SKIN

Deeply coloured fruits, vegetables and herbs are rich in powerful antioxidant carotenoids such as lutein, beta-carotene, lycopene and alpha-lipoeic acid. The denser the colour, the higher the antioxidant content. Try incorporating these top-ten antioxidant-rich fruit and vegetables into your diet:

Avocado High in fibre and monounsaturated fats, they help to enrich the skin from within; rich in antioxidants.

Carrots Full of antioxidant Vitamins A, C and E; contain high levels of beta-carotene which promotes healthy digestion and protects against cancer; cleanses the liver and the blood.

Sweet potatoes Packed full of beta-carotene and vitamin C; rich in fibre.

Squash Good source of beta-carotene and Vitamin C.

Broccoli High in antioxidants including Vitamin C and the Vitamin A precursor beta-carotene; a good source of fibre.

Tomato Contains antioxidant Vitamins C and E, and beta-carotene.

Apricots High levels of beta-carotene, which the body turns into Vitamin A.

Citrus fruit Oranges, lemons and grapefruits are all high in vitamin C and other antioxidants.

Apple Apples have been found to have very strong antioxidant activity.

Other ingredients that help keep skin nourished and moisturised from the inside include grains like millet (rich in mineral salt and silicon, which mends and aids elimination of toxins) and quinoa (high in protein and essential minerals); the essential fatty acids found in oily fish like mackerel and sardines, and in the oil and seeds of flax, pumpkin, almonds and hemp.

Chapter 2

Preservatives and Colours

Preservatives

Preservatives, by their very nature, are designed to kill things. Specifically they work by killing cells and preventing them from multiplying and are intended to inhibit the growth of bacteria and fungi – what most of us just call 'germs' – in commercial products. These germs include *Candida albicans*, *Pseudomonas aeruginosa*, *Escherechia coli*, *Aspergillus niger* and *Stephylococcus aureus* – which can potentially cause serious infections on the skin and in the body.

No preservative will completely prevent these contaminants from getting into the products you use – the purpose of a preservative is simply to keep their growth in the bottle, tube or tub to a minimum.

Bacteria and fungi can get into personal-care products in several ways. Product formulators commonly put the blame on consumers for introducing germs into a product with use – for instance by dipping unwashed hands into tubs, leaving tops off, diluting with water, storing in a warm, moist bathroom, buying large, wide-mouth containers that the entire family can and does use. But a significant amount of contamination actually occurs during manufacture – a problem that should be, but is rarely, addressed at the level of factory-floor hygiene instead of simply adding more chemicals to the finished product.

Finding new preservatives for cosmetic formulators is complicated because, in order to be considered effective, a preservative has to fulfil several criteria. It must be:

- Effective across a wide range of microbes
- Long lasting (continues to keep the product free from contaminants for the life of the product)
- Rapid acting at the first sign of contamination
- Non-sensitising (doesn't produce allergic reactions)
- Non-toxic and non-irritating
- Compatible with the other ingredients in the mix
- Stable (not break down during storage and stays active in a wide pH range)
- Inactive, except as an anti-microbial (not interact with other ingredients)
- Soluble (mixes well with whatever base (water or oil) it is in)
- Acceptable in odour and colour
- Cost effective

No single preservative, synthetic or natural, fulfils all these criteria, which is one reason why manufacturers often use mixtures of several different preservatives in a single product. Another reason is solubility; some preservatives are water-soluble and some are oil-soluble. For products that contain both water and oil (see p. 31 for more), such as a hand lotion, formulators need to use both types of preservative.

Like pesticides, preservatives are designed to kill living things. Widespread concern about the use of cosmetic preservatives stems from the fact that human skin is a living organ comprised of living cells. Preservatives, even if they are used in small quantities, present a risk to the integrity of the skin and, should they be absorbed into the bloodstream, to the rest of the body. For this reason most cosmetic preservatives generally have restrictions on their use – usually limiting them to a small percentage of the total formula.

The worst offenders

All the most commonly used preservatives can cause dermatitis and other skin reactions such as dry, itchy, red or blotchy skin; some pose more risks than others. For instance, the most commonly used cosmetic preservatives belong to a family of chemicals called *alkyl hydroxy benzoates* and are known as parabens. Look on any ingredient label and the chances are you will find *methylparaben, ethylparaben, butylparaben* and *propylparaben* either singly or more often in combination.

Parabens are universally recognised as skin sensitisers (they have the potential to cause an allergic response). In 1998 British researchers published a study that identified parabens as oestrogen mimics as well, each with a different oestrogenic potency. *Methylparaben* was the least potent, followed by *ethylparaben, propylparaben* and finally *butylparaben.* Oestrogen mimics are a concern because even in small amounts they can disrupt the normal hormone balance of the body. Like many other oestrogen mimics parabens have also been linked to cancer. In studies of breast tumours, traces of parabens have been found in every single sample, suggesting that this oestrogenic effect is not just confined to the lab.

After parabens, *Kathon CG* – the main constituents of which are *methylisochlorothiazolinone* and *methylchlorothiazolinone* – is the most common preservative ingredient in cosmetics. Like parabens, it is a common allergen and sensitiser (that is to say, over time even small amounts can cause sensitivity reactions).

Although they are widely used in cosmetics today, a study conducted more than a decade ago found that *Kathon CG* was also 'mutagenic' – in other words capable of causing genetic mutations. This study was the first to test commercially available products containing this preservative, and the researchers noted that when a product is both a sensitiser and a mutagen it also has the potential to cause cancer and that 'more adequate testing for its cancer-causing potential is needed.' Since then, laboratory studies have found that *methylisochlorothiazolinone* is also a neurotoxin, that is to say it is toxic to your nervous system (which controls various body functions such as heartbeat and breathing) as well as affecting mood and memory.

LIFTING THE LID

Between 10 and 30 per cent of adults experience skin problems from exposure to preservatives and fragrances in cosmetic products.

Natural preservatives

While the idea of a 'preservative-free' product sounds good, there is no such thing. All commercial products require some degree of preservation and while products based on plant extracts, for instance, may claim to be preservative-free this is often because the active plant ingredients also function as preservatives.

With natural preservatives such as essential oils, herbal and fruit extracts, sugars and even grains, the shelf life of the product may be shorter and the overall package may need to be smaller, but the trade-off is better skin health in the short term and better overall health over the longer term.

In studies of breast tumours, traces of parabens have been found in every single sample

Reduce your exposure to potentially toxic preservatives by buying plant-based products in smaller containers. Products that are hermetically sealed or provide a metered-dose (i.e. pumps and squeeze tops) allow fewer contaminants during storage and so require fewer preservatives. Likewise collapsible tubes discourage contamination, which is why they are so widely used in pharmaceuticals. Tubes made from aluminium have a preservative effect and they are recyclable.

The following botanicals can often be used as both active ingredients and effective natural preservatives:

- Aloe vera
- Citrus seed extract
- Clove
- Cranberry extract
- Cypress
- Eucalyptus
- Lavender
- Manuka
- Neem (fast-growing evergreen)
- Propolis (tree resin)
- Rose
- Rosemary
- Sage
- Sandalwood
- Tea tree
- Thyme
- Willow bark
- Witch hazel
- Yerba mansa (hardy perennial)
- Yucca

Because there are few profits to be made from truly natural preservatives, many companies are formulating patented blends of so-called 'natural' preservatives, which they advertise on the label as natural preservative 'systems'. Some are more natural than others and it's always worth checking with the manufacturer what's actually in the 'system' before accepting that it is 'natural'.

Colours

It starts when you get up in the morning. You grab a bar of soap or a bottle of shower foam and you have a wash. That's probably your first dip into the daily palette of synthetic tints and hues that will colour much of your day.

Contact with cosmetic colours is a 24/7 experience that includes multiple exposures to multiple products. Regulatory authorities and cosmetics manufacturers go to great lengths to assure us that these colour additives are safe and add an important feel-good factor to their products; but there is little objective scientific evidence that this is the case.

SKIN REACTIONS

If you find that your skin reacts quickly to the products you use it might be worth avoiding those that contain the following preservatives:

- Benzoic acid
- BHT (butylated hydroxytoulene)
- Butylparaben
- C12-15 alkyl benzoate
- Diazolidinyl urea
- Disodium EDTA
- EDTA
- Ethylparaben
- Formaldehyde
- Isobutylparaben
- Methylchloroisothiazolinone
- Methylisothiazolinone
- Methylparaben
- Phenoxyethanol
- Propylparaben
- Quaternium 15
- Salicylic acid
- Sodium benzoate
- Sorbic acid
- Tetrasodium EDTA

While a single use of a single coloured product may be 'safe', your total daily exposure to all the artificially coloured products – soaps, body lotions, shampoos, conditioners, shaving cream, toothpaste, deodorants, hair dyes, lipsticks, eye shadows and blushers – may add up to an unacceptable risk.

Colours used in cosmetics generally fall into one of three categories: organic, inorganic and natural.

Organic colours are derived primarily from petroleum and are sometimes known as coal-tar dyes or synthetic-organic colours. Inorganic colours include clays, iron oxides (which can produce yellows, browns, blacks, reds) and ultramarines (including chromium oxide green, mica, titanium dioxide, zinc oxide and kaolin clay).

Reduce your exposure to potentially toxic preservatives by buying plant-based products in smaller containers

Although they can be derived from earth sources, inorganic colours are not generally considered natural because they are heat treated to various temperatures to produce different colours. Some like mica can be coated with organic colours to give them a particular hue.

Furthermore, whereas many oxides and ultramarines used to be mined, due to today's concerns about purity (mined products can be contaminated with lead, arsenic, mercury, antimony and selenium) many of these colourants are manufactured in a lab.

Natural colours are those that are derived from or that come directly from plant or animal sources.

Checking for the presence of potentially harmful dyes in cosmetics is difficult because even within the same country, a colour can be listed on the label under any number of different names. In Europe colours are usually listed by their INCI (International Nomenclature for Cosmetic Ingredients) numbers – usually the prefix CI followed by five numbers. In the US, the same colours are listed with FD&C (Foods, Drugs and Dosmetics) prefixes or with a D&C (Drugs and Cosmetics) prefix.

Another worry is that the experts cannot agree on an international safe list of colours. Some colours may be allowed in one country, but banned elsewhere. Some cosmetic colours are known to cause problems in susceptible individuals.

Most organic colours, for instance, can cause skin irritation; some can block pores. Even inorganic mineral pigments, which are generally considered safer than petroleum-derived colours, can and do produce sensitivity reactions like skin rashes. Iron oxides, for example, which are commonly used in make-up, contain the irritant nickel. A significant percentage of the population – around 18 per cent – is allergic to nickel.

More worrying is the fact that many commonly used organic colours have been shown to cause cancerous growths on the skins of animals which could be as a result of the raw materials used to make them or because of the presence of carcinogenic impurities in some batches.

Banned carcinogenic colours regularly appear in cosmetics that have been illegally imported from abroad

The colour con

New colours are being developed all the time, but this is not always necessarily with an eye on safety. One of the newest, FD&C red 40 (also known as Allura Red or CI16035) is a popular addition to eyeshadows. It has been in use since 1994 despite the fact that all the safety testing was funded and performed by the manufacturer, rather

LIFTING THE LID

Colour serves no practical purpose in body-care products, though its psychological impact is an important sales incentive. Manufacturers use colour to link the product to an emotion or state of mind. Thus a pink product will be perceived as soft and girlish, which is why it is so often found in products for teenagers and, ironically, 'mature' women. A light green might indicate freshness while white or blue are linked with purity and sensitivity.

than an independent body. The National Cancer Institute in the US reports that *p-credine*, a chemical used in the manufacturing of FD&C red 40, is a carcinogen.

There is simply not enough evidence to prove how safe any cosmetic colours are on the skin with long-term use. If you absolutely must have a coloured product, check the label for colour additives beginning CI75- as these are 'natural', usually vegetable-based, colourants (see list, p. 24), though some can be highly synthesised. Those beginning with CI77- are inorganic colours that may be somewhat safer than their organic cousins. If you want to use safer products, though, the most effective thing you can do is choose products that are not coloured at all. Alternatively, try to avoid those that contain the colours in the following table:

Common name	Europe	US
Alizarine Cyanine Green F	CI61570	D&C Green 5
Acetate Blue G	CI64500	Disperese Blue 1
Acetate Fast Yellow	CI11855	Disperese Yellow 3
Acid Red 33	CI17200	D&C Red 33
Allura Red	CI16035	FD&C Red 40
Brilliant Blue FCF	CI42090	FD&C Blue 1
Fast Green FCF	CI42053	FD&C Green 3
Indigo Carmine	CI73015	FD&C Blue 2
Pigment Orange 5	CI12075	D&C Orange 17
Pigment Red 53 barium salt	CI15585	D&C Red 9
Pigment Red 53 sodium salt	CI15585	D&C Red 8
Ponceau SX	CI14700	FD&C Red 4
Rhodamine B	CI45170	D&C Red 19
Sunset Yellow	CI15985	FD&C Yellow 6
Tartrazine	CI19140	FD&C Yellow 5
Titanium Dioxide	CI77891	Pigment White 6

Certain carcinogenic colours are now banned from use in US and European cosmetics. These include D&C Red 2, 3, 4, 10 and 17, FD&C Red 10 and FD&C Blue 4. Nevertheless, these colours still regularly appear in cosmetics that have been illegally imported from other countries.

Natural substances can be used to colour products and, like natural preservatives, some have multiple functions in the product. If you are looking for products that use natural pigments, look for these ingredients on the label:

- Alfalfa
- Alkanet root oil
- Annatto
- Beetroot
- Bentonite clay
- Beta carotene
- Blue chamomile
- Calendula petals
- Caramel
- Carmine
- Carrot oil extract
- Chlorophyll
- Cocoa powder
- Grape juice
- Henna
- Kelp
- Red cabbage
- Turmeric

While preservatives serve a useful function in cosmetics, colours are there for little more than a feel-good factor. Both can be based on cheap, poorly tested ingredients and the formulator's choice of chemical is often based around what everyone else in the marketplace is doing. Innovative natural products are rarely coloured and the manufacturers of these kinds of toiletries think holistically about the product and its package, for instance using things like airtight packaging, or collapsible aluminium tubes (aluminium has a preservative effect and the collapsible tube keeps the product from going off.) The end result is a better product with fewer potential allergens.

Chapter 3

Detergents and Penetration Enhancers

Body washes, shampoos, bath foams, baby wash and shower gels, facial washes and scrubs – all the foamy stuff we use in the bathroom – rely on complex modern detergents to do the relatively uncomplicated job of cleaning.

Detergents are part of a larger group of chemicals called surfactants (short for 'surface active agents'). Surfactants change the basic properties of water, for instance lowering its surface tension, making it 'wetter' and better able to interact with other additives in the mixture. Detergents have similar properties and can, in addition, add foaming ability.

Common detergents used in cosmetics are also used in industry for degreasing engines

Foam, of course, does nothing to improve the product's cleaning ability. However, manufacturers constantly add more detergent and additional foam boosters to produce the foam that they believe consumers can't live without. This increased concentration of detergent creates the need for other additives such as skin and hair conditioners to counteract some of the harshness of the detergent, generating a much more complex cocktail of ingredients in the attempt to limit any skin reaction to the detergents.

Anionic detergents are the most common detergents used in cosmetics and bodycare. They are popular with manufacturers because they work quickly and effectively in both hard and soft water and they foam and rinse well. But anionic detergents such as *lauryl sulphates*, *sarcosines* and *sulfosuccinates* can also be harsh – so much so that they are prized in industry for heavy-duty clean-ups like degreasing engines. Is this really what you want to be putting on your skin?

Anionic detergents meet all the performance and aesthetic requirements of product formulators and while a detergent on its own is unlikely to be directly toxic, a harsh detergent can strip the skin and hair of protective oils, increasing the risk of dry skin and the absorption of other chemicals into the bloodstream (see 'penetration enhancers', p. 28).

Detergents can be harmful in other indirect ways. Some, especially those with names ending in 'eth' (as in *sodium laureth sulphate*), can be contaminated with the carcinogen *1,4-dioxane*. Others such as *diethanolamine* (*DEA*) can interact with other ingredients in the mix to form cancer-causing substances known as nitrosamines – the same carcinogens found in cigarettes and cured meats.

DEA and its related compounds such as *triethanolamine* (*TEA*) and *monoethanolamine* (*MEA*) can invariably be found in products that foam including bubble bath, body washes, shampoos, soaps and facial cleansers.

Once added to the product these chemicals readily react with any nitrites present to form a compound called *N-nitrosodiethanolamine* (*NDELA*). Nitrites are known cancer-causing substances (see Appendix 1) which can get into personal-care products as contaminants present in raw materials. They can also be the result of additives such as formaldehyde-releasing or formaldehyde-containing chemicals such as *2-bromo-2-nitropropane-1,3-diol* (also known as *BNPD* or *Bronopol*) and *Padimate-O* (*octyl dimethyl PABA*), *DMDM hydantoin*, *diazolidinyl urea*, *imidazolindinyl urea* and *quaternium 15*, so look out for these chemicals in the list of ingredients when you are shopping for replacement products.

Stored for extended periods at elevated temperatures, nitrites will continue to form in a product, and surveys in the US and Europe have shown that between 42 and 93 per cent of all detergent-based products contain nitrosamines.

The alternative

Soap is a simple, effective and largely natural cleanser. Detergents on the other hand can only be produced synthetically and the damage they can do to skin, hair, eyes and mucous membranes varies according to how harsh and denaturing they are. If you are determined to buy detergent-based body-care products you can make safer choices by choosing those made with ingredients that have a milder action on the skin and/or which don't contain potential carcinogens.

As a general rule, try to avoid products that contain the following detergents and surfactants:

- *Ammonium laureth sulphate*
- *Ammonium lauryl sulphate*
- *Cocamide DEA*
- *Cocamide MEA*
- *Cocamidopropyl betaine*
- *DEA olet-3 phosphate*
- *DEA-cetyl phosphate*
- *Diethanolamine (DEA) lauryl sulphate*
- *Glyceryl laurate*
- *Lauramide DEA*
- *Linoleamide MEA*
- *Monoethanolamine (MEA) lauryl sulphate*
- *Myristamide DEA*
- *Oleamide DEA*
- *Sodium laureth sulphate*
- *Sodium lauryl sulphate*
- *Stearamide MEA*
- *Triethanolamine (TEA) lauryl sulphate*

No matter what you see on the label, there is no such thing as a 'natural' detergent. All of them consist of highly processed ingredients whipped up in a lab. Vegetable-based detergents aren't necessarily milder than others, though their environmental impact is somewhat less. Products making use of the mildest detergents use the following ingredients:

- *Amphoteric-2*
- *Amphoteric-20*
- *Amphoteric-6*
- *Cocamidopropyl hydroxysultaine*
- *Cocoa betaine*
- *Cocoa glucoside*
- *Decyl glucose*
- *Decyl polyglucose*
- *Lauryl betaine*
- *Lauryl glucoside*
- *Polysorbate 20*
- *Polysorbate 40*
- *Sodium cocoyl isethionate*
- *Sodium lauraminopropionate*
- *Sorbitan laurate*
- *Sorbitan palmate*
- *Sorbitan stearate*

Penetration enhancers

Most people think of the skin as a barrier. In reality it is more like a sponge and it can quickly absorb a significant amount – scientists estimate up to 60 per cent – of whatever you put onto it.

But the job of estimating how quickly a body-care product penetrates the skin and how deeply it is absorbed depends on a number of factors and is made more complicated by the fact that certain chemicals can speed up the penetration and absorption of others. These ingredients, known as penetration enhancers, are found in all kinds of body-care products, but are particularly widely used in body lotions and face creams.

Penetration-enhancing chemicals have been used to effectively deliver drugs – for instance via hormone and nicotine patches – deeper and faster through the skin and into the blood vessels. The concern when used in cosmetics is not so much that these penetration enhancers are toxic – many of them are safe used on their own – but in the way that they alter the top protective layer of skin (for instance by removing its protective oily layer) in a way that allows other chemicals, which may be more toxic, to be absorbed.

In body-care products, chemicals that act like penetration enhancers usually have more than one function. Often they are major active ingredients like moisturisers, detergents and solvents that are added to moisturise and cleanse. However, they are also deliberately added to products because their penetration-enhancing effects are essential for today's quick-fix products that offer visible but temporary results in under an hour.

Because they dissolve or get past the normally protective oily layer of the skin, penetration enhancers are also significant sources of skin irritation. Using several products laced with these types of ingredients is likely to lead to allergic reactions – for instance, to active ingredient such as fragrances, surfactants and preservatives – in people with susceptible skins. In one American study, over 10 per cent of the allergic reactions studied were due to the effect of penetration-enhancing emollients.

Moisturising, or emollient, ingredients can include any oil or fatty acid – anything that makes the product 'creamy' – but these days also include liposomes and nanosomes, which are microscopic emollients designed specifically to be small enough to get through the skin's normal filters and drive ingredients into the deeper layers of skin.

Many solvents, for instance ingredients that have *PEG* in their name, are used as penetration enhancers. These, as well as perfumes and the detergents used in shampoos and shower gels, alter the structure of the skin by dissolving its protective oily barrier, and in this way allow other chemicals in the mix to penetrate more deeply into the skin. Because the upper layers of the skin are criss-crossed with tiny blood vessels, these chemicals will also eventually find their way into your bloodstream and your internal organs.

The list of ingredients that can act as penetration enhancers is incredibly long but it commonly includes:

- **Solvents** such as acetone, ethanol, limonene, *polyethylene glycol (PEG), propylene glycol (PPG), xylene, acetamide* and *trichloroethanol*.
- **Fatty acid esters** such as *butyl acetate, diethyl succinate, ethyl acetate,* and some *isopropyl, methyl* and *sorbitan* compounds.
- **Fatty acids** such as capric acid, lactic acid, linoleic acid, linolenic acid, oleaic acid and palmitic acid.
- **Ionic compounds** such as ionic surfactants, *sodium lauryl sulphate, sodium carboxylate, sodium hyaluronate* and *sodium ascorbate*.
- **Complexing agents** such as *lipsomes, naphthalene,* classical and nonionic surfactants and *nonoxynol*.

How much you absorb from a particular product will also depend on the condition of your skin. This in turn is can be a reflection of the number and types of products you use every day. For instance, a body wash based on harsh detergents may strip the skin of protective oils. If you then apply a moisturiser with a range of penetration enhancers in it, the chances are those ingredients will get much deeper into your skin than if you had bathed with a gentler soap and used a simpler moisturiser.

Detergents and penetration enhancers, while not necessarily dangerous in themselves, can make the skin more permeable to other chemicals. For this reason it is worthwhile questioning the number of products we use and buy which foam and fizz as well as those promising quick-fix results. As the advice in Part 2 shows there are many better ways to get clean and have great skin that don't involve waging chemical warfare on your skin.

Chapter 4

Moisturisers and Emulsifiers

Moisturisers perform a very basic function in maintaining the water balance in the uppermost layers of the skin. This area of the skin, known as the *stratum corneum*, is made up of cells that are constantly shed and replaced by new cells emerging from the deeper layers of the skin. The *stratum corneum* contains approximately 30 per cent water. Two thirds of this is bound to biological tissues and this does not usually change unless you are suffering from a serious skin condition such as eczema or psoriasis. But the remaining water content rises and falls according to what's going on in your environment, for instance dry weather conditions, over-washing or exposure to central heating, air conditioning and certain chemicals.

Moisturising ingredients work in two ways to help slow this water loss. Humectants such as *propylene glycol* and urea act like water magnets, drawing moisture from the atmosphere and keeping it near the skin.

Emollients are generally fats, oils and waxes that form a barrier on the surface of the skin. For years, moisturising creams and lotions relied on emollients like the mineral oil lanolin to provide this protective barrier. Today, synthetic derivatives of vegetable oils such as *isopropyl palmitate* and *hexyl laureate* are more common, as are a range of synthetic 'film formers' such as silicone and *PTFE* (Teflon).

Do they work?

Moisturisers are generally mixtures of oil and water (or 'emulsions', see p. 32). To keep these two opposing substances bound together, and to make sure the product has a long shelf life, a cream or lotion will contain a raft of emulsifiers, stabilizers and preservatives. To make it more pleasant to use it will also contain perfumes and colours. If the cream also claims other properties such as improving wrinkles, further ingredients are added.

So what starts out as a simple emulsion quickly becomes a cocktail of harmful ingredients. And here's the catch: the emollients also act like penetration enhancers – ingredients that aid the absorption of other more toxic substances into the skin and eventually the blood stream.

Hardly surprising then that moisturising creams can and do cause problems like allergic reactions, skin irritation and contact dermatitis, all characterised by redness, itching, burning and stinging sensations. Used over the long term, they can also create the very problem they are intended to solve by actually increasing water loss from the skin.

Toxic ingredients

Some moisturising ingredients, however, are harmful in their own right. Mineral oil, a by-product of the distillation of gasoline from crude oil, impedes the skin's ability to breathe, attract moisture and detoxify. It can also slow down cell renewal and promote premature skin ageing. Any mineral oil derivative can be contaminated with cancer-causing *polycyclic aromatic hydrocarbons (PAHs)*.

Mineral oil used in moisturisers can slow down cell renewal and promote premature skin ageing

Humectants such as *alpha hydroxy acids* (lactic acid or glycolic acid) act like chemical peels, thinning the *stratum corneum* and ultimately accelerating water loss. Many emollients trap dirt and sweat under the skin, some like *petrolatum* degrade the skin's natural protective barrier which makes it more vulnerable to bacteria and viruses.

Film-forming ingredients like *PTFE* (Teflon) and *dimethicone* are now routinely added to cosmetics and body-care products without any comprehensive evaluation of their safety. Teflon contains the potential carcinogen *PFOA* and some silicones are known tumour promoters which accumulate in the liver and lymph nodes. Both are non-biodegradable.

Newer moisturisers are already using nanoparticles that slip into the spaces between skin cells before releasing their active ingredients. No research has been conducted to show how much more of these substances is absorbed into the blood stream, so if you want to avoid them, look for words like 'liposome' or 'nanosome' on the label. If you wish to avoid using synthetic moisturisers watch out for the following ingredients on the label:

- *Acrylates/C10-30 alkyl acrylate crosspolymer*
- *Cyclomethicone*
- *Cyclopentasiloxane*
- *Decyl oleate*
- *Dimethicone*
- *Dimethicone copolyol*
- *Dioctyl cyclohexane*
- *Hexyl decanol*
- *Hexyl laureate*
- *Isopropyl myristate*
- *Isopropyl palmitate*
- *Isopropyl stearate*
- *Octyl dodecanol*
- *Oleyl alcohol*
- *Paraffinum liquidum*
- *Petrolatum*
- *Propylene glycol*
- *Simethicone*
- Lactic acid
- Glycolic acid
- Urea

Emulsifiers

Many of the ingredients in commercial toiletries are uneasy bedfellows; none more so than water and oil. Anybody who has ever made a salad dressing or a sauce knows these two don't combine well unless you add something else – such as salt or mustard. Emulsifiers are essentially the glue that holds incompatible ingredients together, producing a stable, homogeneous product with an even texture that formulators call an emulsion. An emulsifier can either be a physical substance (like a wax), which will generally hold the ingredients in suspension indefinitely, or a physical action such as the instruction to shake well before use.

For the purposes of understanding toiletries there are two basic types of emulsions:

- **Oil in Water** – In this emulsion water is the dominant ingredient. Oil in water emulsions are used to create cream and lotions that feel moist and less greasy. When absorbed into the skin there is very little to no oily residue.
- **Water in Oil** – In this emulsion oil is the dominant ingredient. You will find this mixture in heavier creams, and those used to treat rough skin. The level of greasiness depends on the formula – all of which will be absorbed into the skin, albeit more slowly.

NATURAL MOISTURISERS

Look or these natural ingredients when choosing natural products:

- Almond oil
- Aloe vera
- Apricot kernel oil
- Avocado oil
- Beeswax
- Castor oil
- Cocoa butter
- Coconut oil
- Emu oil*
- Evening primrose oil
- Glycerine
- Grapeseed oil
- Hemp seed oil
- Honey
- Jojoba
- Macadamia nut oil
- Mango butter
- Olive oil
- Rosa mosqueta oil
- Shea butter
- Squalene
- Wheatgerm oil

When you are buying natural alternatives to conventional moisturisers, remember to look for these natural oils on the label, and to buy those products that have the fewest ingredients. It is also worth remembering that even though manufacturers tell you that you should moisturise every day, this is not necessariy so. It is good to give your skin a break from having anything on it. Moisturise when you need to, and if you skin seems ok, give it a day off from products.

*Most of these are plant based. Emu oil is an animal based oil which is a by-product of emu meat production. Very similar in structure to human sebum, it can be very soothing on very dry skin.

A CHEMICAL-FREE ALTERNATIVE

Emulsifiers are only necessary if you make a product that mixes oil and water. So the real question might be: do we need oil- and water-based products? Often the answer is no. In the case of moisturisers, you can use single oils (such as jojoba or rosehip) to keep your skin supple. These are best applied onto damp skin or with damp hands to ease their application and to stop you from using too much and feeling greasy. Applying oil or an oil-based moisturiser in this way effectively does the same job as applying an oil/water mixture, without the extra chemicals.

Many toiletries, including creams, lotions, toothpastes, soaps and various other cosmetics, contain emulsifiers. Although they are generally minor ingredients in any product, they confer no real benefit to the skin. Often they are used in conjunction with solubilisers – solvents that keep other ingredients in the mix dissolved. Complex blends of ingredients typically aren't stable for more than a few days without emulsifiers and solubilisers. Without them the oil and water would separate and other ingredients would drop to the bottom or float to the top of the bottle.

Those who question the use of emulsifiers are often labelled as puritans. After all, how can we make great-looking and feeling products without them? In fact very few manufacturers – even those that purport to make natural toiletries – regard emulsifiers as a problem. But because these ingredients simply address aesthetics and ease-of-use issues, it's worth at least pausing to consider both their safety and necessity.

Many types of body-care products, for instance, make use of *polyethylene glycol* (*PEG*) compounds, which are derived from the petrochemical gases ethylene and propylene. They belong to a large family of chemicals that among their many other uses, can be effective emulsifiers. They can also irritate sensitive or damaged skin and have been associated with kidney damage in animals.

According to one report, impurities found in various *PEG*

compounds include *ethylene oxide* and *1,4-dioxane* (both human carcinogens); *polycyclic* aromatic compounds; and heavy metals such as lead, iron, cobalt, nickel, cadmium and the notorious poison arsenic.

In spite of this, the cosmetics industry believes that *PEGs* are generally 'safe for use' in cosmetics but should 'not be used on damaged skin'. Because of this, *PEGs* continue to be used in body-care products, though their presence on the label would indicate a product that it best avoided.

Sometimes surfactants (see p. 25) double as emulsifiers. An example of this is *triethanolamine* (*TEA*, often used as a pH balancer) which can sometimes cause severe allergic reactions, dry skin and eye problems, and can become a sensitiser with prolonged use. Mixed with formaldehyde-forming ingredients such as the preservatives *2-bromo-2-nitropropane-1,3-diol DMDM hydantoin, diazolidinyl urea, imidazolindinyl urea* and *quaternium 15, TEA* can promote the formation of cancer-causing substances known as nitrosamines (see 'Detergents', p. 25).

Searching for emulsifiers on the label can be a bit of a minefield. Some such as emulsifying wax sound more natural than they are. Emulsifying wax, for example, is label shorthand for an ingredient made from other largely synthetic ingredients including: *polysorbate 60, PEG-150 stearate* (which can be animal or vegetable in origin) and *steareth-20* – all three of which can be contaminated with the carcinogen *1,4-dioxane*. Others such as *decyl glucoside*, which can be made from cornstarch, are effective natural emulsifiers, but are not available as organic ingredients.

When selecting products, consider avoiding synthetic emulsifiers:

- *Carbomer*
- *Carboxymethylcellulose*
- *Ceresin (Mineral wax, Ozokerite)*
- *Diethanolamine (DEA)*
- *Isopropyl stearate (laurate, palmitate, oleate, etc.)*
- *PEG compounds (e.g. PEG-8 myristate, PEG-30 glyceryl cocoate, PEG-80 glyceryl cocoate PEG 15 soyamide/IPDI copolymer, PEG-40 sorbitan peroleate, PEG-150 stearate)*
- *Polysorbate 20*
- *Polysorbate 60*
- *Polysorbate 80*

- *Potassium hydroxide*
- *Propylene glycol*
- *Sorbitan stearate (laurate, palmitate, oleate etc)*
- *Steareth-20*
- *Triethanolamine (TEA)*

There are excellent alternatives. Many manufacturers are now making good use of more natural emulsifiers like:

- Beeswax
- Candelilla
- Carnauba
- Cetearyl alcohol
- Cetearyl wheat bran glycosides
- Cetearyl wheat straw glycosides
- *Decyl glucoside*

- Jojoba
- Lecithin
- Quince seed
- Rice bran wax
- Sucrose cocoate
- Vegetable glycerin
- Xanthan gum

Switching over to products that are based on pure oils and waxes will solve two beauty problems in one go. First of all they are better for your skin (and you need to use less to get the same results), and secondly they will almost certainly eliminate the need for an emulsifier which might potentially contain unwanted contaminants.

LIFTING THE LID

In fact, none of the current emulsifiers – even the natural ones – are currently available in organic form, which is why the seal of the UK's organic certification body, the Soil Association, cannot be found on products that appear to be emulsions of natural ingredients. Other organic certification bodies are less strict so as always it's worth paying attention to what the label actually says. For instance, is the whole product certified organic or just some of its ingredients? In the UK at least, choosing Soil Association certified organic products can eliminate a whole host of concerns you might have about emulsifiers at a stroke, and uncomplicate your life enormously.

Chapter 5
Fragrances

Counting up the variety of perfumed body-care products we use on a daily basis can be quite a surprise: soaps, creams and body lotions, ointments, talc and bubble baths, shampoos, sunscreens – to name just a few.

In an overcrowded market, where there is often little to differentiate the performance of one product over another, a product's scent is its unique signature and is frequently given greater prominence in advertising than performance.

Our love affair with perfume has a long history. For many centuries perfumes were made from natural plant and animal sources. But these can be expensive and subject to the variations of season and availability. With scientific progress, manufacturers found ways of producing chemicals with 'nature identical' smells which could be made in vast quantities without worrying about the scarcity of natural resources. Today, nearly all fragrance chemicals are synthesised almost entirely from petrochemicals, and while they can be made more cheaply and the scent may linger longer than that of a naturally derived scents, they are problematical for human health.

Today we use them on our bodies, on our pets, on our children, on our furniture, on our clothes and on most of the surfaces in our homes. Our attitude to fragrance has allowed advertisers to pull the wool over consumers' eyes by linking fragrance with desirable qualities such as love, sexiness, freshness, innocence or even a wild, independent spirit. This message is so persuasive that some individuals feel they can't be attractive unless they are wearing a scent. Our belief in the transformative power of scent has even led us to put faith in products that promise some sort life-changing aromatherapy for the home.

Fragrances add little to the function of the product. They are unlikely to provide the 'aromatherapy' experience promised, especially if they are synthetic. Nevertheless, the way things smell is a tactic used in the marketing of all body-care products, and to particularly great effect in fine perfumes – just consider how many are named after emotions.

The word parfum belies the hundreds of ingredients involved in producing a single scent

The addition of 'parfum' (in the EU) or 'fragrance' (in the USA) is a particularly thorny issue for consumers because most of us will never know which fragrance chemicals are in the products we use. Manufacturers are allowed to simply list them under simple shorthand names which belie the often hundreds of different ingredients that are involved in producing a single scent (even the simplest fragrances are made up of between 30 and 50 ingredients). First and foremost, many of these chemicals are considered hazardous waste. As far back as 1986, the US National Academy of Sciences identified fragrance ingredients as one of six categories of neurotoxic chemicals that should be thoroughly investigated for their potential harm to human health. This placed these chemicals right up there with insecticides, heavy metals, solvents and food additives as primary causes of disease in humans. Government and industry, however, have been slow to demand or fund such research.

Inhaled fragrance chemicals can cause a sore throat, a runny nose, sinus congestion, wheezing, shortness of breath, nausea and muscle pain. They are also a major trigger of asthmatic episodes. Studies have also shown that inhaling fragrance chemicals can cause circulatory changes in the brain and changes in its electrical activity. These changes can result in symptoms like headache, mental confusion, listlessness, inability to concentrate, irritability, seizures, restlessness, agitation, depression and sleepiness. At least one study has demonstrated links between heavy perfume exposure during pregnancy and learning disabilities and behaviour disorders in children.

FRAGRANCE REACTIONS

Once in the body, fragrance chemicals can easily breach the blood-brain barrier – the protective membrane designed to keep toxins away from sensitive brain cells – and produce symptoms of central nervous system (CNS) disruption. Studies have shown that chronic problems associated with exposure to fragrance chemicals include:

- Agitation
- Anaphylaxis
- Anxiety
- Asthma
- Bronchitis
- Confusion
- Coughing
- Depression
- Difficulty breathing
- Difficulty swallowing
- Disorientation
- Dizziness
- Double vision
- Ear pain
- Eczema
- Fatigue
- Flushing
- Headaches
- Hives
- Hypertension
- Incoherence

- Irregular heart beat
- Irritability
- Laryngitis
- Lethargy
- Mood swings
- Muscle/joint pain
- Muscle weakness
- Nasal congestion
- Nausea
- Poor concentration
- Rashes
- Restlessness
- Seizures
- Short-term memory loss
- Sinusitis
- Sneezing
- Spaciness
- Swollen lymph glands
- Tinnitus
- Vertigo
- Watery or dry eyes

Fragrance chemicals are implicated in longer-term health problems as well. Because they are largely made from neurotoxic solvents – many of which have been labelled as toxic waste by the American Food and Drug Administration (FDA) – a lifetime of use may contribute to central nervous system (CNS) disorders such as multiple sclerosis, Parkinson's disease and Alzheimer's disease. Heavy use of fragranced products is also associated with higher rates of sudden infant death syndrome (SIDS).

In addition to being inhaled, fragrances can be absorbed through the skin. Children's skin, which is thinner than that of adults, is especially vulnerable. The creamier the product you are using (think skin creams, roll-on deodorants) the greater the absorbency. While fragrance chemicals can be quick to saturate the blood, they are slow to clear from the body. When they penetrate the skin they can cause discoloration of internal organs. Some are also toxic to the liver and kidneys. Still others accumulate in fatty tissue and leech slowly back into the system or are passed on to our children through breast milk.

The fragrance portion of a product is responsible for around 15 per cent of all allergic reactions in eczema patients, a trend that is increasing. And while synthetic fragrances are most commonly used and thus most commonly implicated, emerging evidence suggests that natural fragrances can also cause allergic reactions. It's not just adult cosmetics that are a problem, either. Play make-up and perfumes aimed at children often contain unacceptably high levels of these substances too.

According to a US Environmental Protection Agency report, the 20 most common fragrance ingredients make up a toxic soup that few of us would willingly be exposed to. Of these, seven – *1,8-cineole*; *b-citronellol*; *b-myrcene*; *nerol*; *ocimene*; *b-phenethyl alcohol*; *a-terpinolene* – are completely lacking in safety data. Of the rest:

- **Acetone** is on the 'hazardous waste' lists of several government agencies. It is primarily a CNS depressant, which means it can cause dryness of the mouth and throat, dizziness, nausea, lack of co-ordination, slurred speech, drowsiness and, in severe exposures, coma.
- **Benzaldehyde** acts as a local anaesthetic and CNS depressant. It can cause irritation to the mouth, throat, eyes, skin, lungs and gastrointestinal tract, causing nausea and abdominal pain. It has also been shown to cause kidney damage.

- *Benzyl acetate* is an environmental pollutant and potential carcinogen linked to pancreatic cancer. Its vapours are irritating to eyes and respiratory passages and it can also be absorbed through the skin causing system-wide effects.

- *Benzyl alcohol* is irritating to the upper respiratory tract. It can cause headache, nausea, vomiting, dizziness, a drop in blood pressure, CNS depression and, in severe cases, death due to respiratory failure.

- **Camphor** is a local irritant and CNS stimulant that is readily absorbed through body tissues. Inhalation can irritate eyes, nose and throat and cause dizziness, confusion, nausea, twitching muscles and convulsions.

- **Ethanol** is on the Environmental Protection Agency (EPA) 'hazardous waste' list. It causes CNS disorders and is irritating to the eyes and upper respiratory tract even in low concentrations. Inhalation of its vapours has the same effects as ingestion. These include an initial stimulatory effect followed by drowsiness, impaired vision, loss of muscle co-ordination and stupor.

- **Ethyl acetate** is on the EPA 'hazardous waste' list. It is a narcotic which is irritating to the eyes and respiratory tract. It can cause headache and stupor. It removes the protective oily barrier of the skin and may cause drying and cracking. In extreme cases it may cause anaemia with leukocytosis (an abnormal and dangerous increase in white blood cells) and damage to liver and kidneys.

- *Limonene* is a carcinogen, a skin and eye irritant and an allergen.

- *Linalool* is a narcotic and causes CNS disorders. It has been shown to cause sometimes fatal respiratory disturbances, poor muscular co-ordination, reduced spontaneous motor activity and depression. Animal tests have shown it may also affect the heart.

- *Methylene chloride* was banned by the FDA in 1988 but no enforcement is possible due to trade secret laws protecting the chemical fragrance industry. It is on the 'hazardous waste' lists of several government agencies. A carcinogen and CNS disrupter, it is absorbed and stored in body fat. It metabolises to carbon monoxide, reducing the oxygen-carrying capacity of the blood so less oxygen gets to the cells, vital organs and the brain. Other adverse effects include headache, giddiness, stupor, irritability, fatigue, tingling in the limbs.

- **A-pinene** is a sensitiser that is damaging to the immune system.

- **G-terpinene** causes asthma and CNS disorders.
- **A-terpineol** is highly irritating to mucous membranes; aspiration into the lungs can produce pneumonitis (inflammation of lung tissue) or even fatal oedema (excess fluid retention) it can also cause nervous excitement, loss of muscular co-ordination, hypothermia, CNS and respiratory depression and headache. Scientific data warns against repeated or prolonged skin contact.

Some perfumes do now list their ingredients on the label. In addition, labelling rules have changed in the last few years and manufacturers' fragranced products of all kinds – including toiletries and household cleaners – must list any of the 26 fragrances that the EU's Scientific Committee on Cosmetic Products and Non-Food Products (SCCNFP) has identified as common contact allergies (see below). So now it's easy enough to avoid these. But the fragrances not listed on the label are still potentially powerful enough to trigger more subtle emotional symptoms or longer-term health problems.

The fragrance chemicals known to cause allergic reactions are:

- *Amyl cinnamal*
- *Amylcinnamyl alcohol*
- *Benzyl alcohol*
- *Benzyl salicylate*
- *Cinnamyl alcohol*
- *Cinnamal*
- *Citral*
- *Coumarin*
- *Eugenol*
- *Geraniol*
- *Hydroxycitronellal*
- *Hydroxymethylpentylcyclohexene carboxaldehyde*
- *Isoeugenol*
- *Anisyl alcohol*
- *Benzyl benzoate*
- *Benzyl cinnamate*
- *Citronellol*
- *Farnesol*
- *Hexylcinnamaldehyde*
- *Lilial (2-(4-tert-butylbenzyl) propionaldehyde)*
- *d-Limonene*
- *Linalool*
- *Methyl heptine carbonate*
- *g-Methylionone (3-methyl-4-(2,6, 6-trimethyl-2-cyclohexen-1-yl)-3-buten-2-one)*
- Oak moss
- Tree moss

But this doesn't mean you can't enjoy scented products. Natural essential oils make a good alternative to synthetic perfumes. Occasionally, these have multiple functions, for instance as an 'active ingredient' (i.e. one that has a beneficial effect on the skin), a preservative and a fragrance.

- Bergamot (*Citrus bergamia*)
- Cedarwood (*Cedrus atlantica*)
- Chamomile (*Anthemis nobilis* or *Chamomilla recutita*)
- Citronella (*Cymbopogon nardus*)
- Frankincense (*Olibanum*)
- Geranium (*Pelargonium graveolens*)
- Jasmine (*Jasmin grandifolium*)
- Lavender (*Lavandula angustifolia*)
- Lemon (*Citrus medica limonum*)
- Mandarin (*Citrus reticulata*)
- Melissa (*Melissa officinalis*)
- Myrrh (*Commiphora myrrha*)
- Neroli (*Citrus aurantium*)
- Palmarose (*Cymbopogon martini*)
- Patchouli (*Pogostemon patchouli*)
- Peppermint (*Mentha piperita*)
- Pettigrain (*Citrus aurantium*)
- Rose (*Rosa centifolia*)
- Rosemary (*Rosmarinus officinalis*)
- Rosewood (*Aniba rosaeodora*)
- Sandalwood (*Santalum album*)
- Sweet orange oil (*Citrus aurantium dulcis*)
- Tea tree (*Melaleuca alternifolia*)
- Ylang ylang (*Cananga odorata genuine*)

Natural fragrances

The list of 'bad' fragrance chemicals on p. 40 contains a large number of substances that are naturally present as constituents of the essential oils listed above. This is because the law requires that 16 naturally occurring fragrance constituents should also be listed on the label because of their allergenic potential. This means that, for example, any product that contains geranium essential oil must also list geraniol on the ingredients list even though it is not added separately, but is merely present as a natural component of the essential oil. So what's the difference?

Very simply it is this: in the matrix of an essential oil there exist substances, some of which have been identified and some of which we have yet to identify, which seem to reduce the potential of an allergic reaction. These co-factors are not present when a substance, such as geraniol or limonene, is extracted and used singly or when it is synthesised in the lab.

When fragrances penetrate the skin they can cause discoloration of internal organs

The European guidelines were drawn up because of the high incidence of reported allergic reactions to these substances. Since 95 per cent of fragrances used in consumer products are synthetic in origin, it is safe to assume that these allergic reactions were largely due to the synthetic forms.

It would have been more helpful to consumers and fairer to

USING ESSENTIAL OILS

Only a very few essential oils are safe to use neat on the skin. The best way to use most oils is to mix them in a base oil, sometimes called a carrier oil. Simple sunflower oil from your kitchen cupboard is as good a choice as any. Other good choices include sweet almond, apricot kernel, grapeseed, safflower and hazelnut oils. To enrich a base oil, try adding heavier oils such as carrot, borage seed, avocado, evening primrose, jojoba, wheatgerm or sesame. Because they are so rich and heavy, these oils should account for no more than 10 per cent of any base mixture.

When mixing your essential oils in the base, the general rule is use no more than 1 drop of essential oil to 1 ml of base oil. A tablespoon of oil equals about 15ml, so you could use up to 15 drops of essential oil. You can mix different essential oils to make your own unique scent, but keep it simple, you probably don't need more than five different oils in a single mixture.

producers of natural products if the guidelines had in some way drawn the distinction between natural and synthetic substances (and such changes are currently being considered). Frustratingly, under current labelling laws there is no way for a consumer to tell which fragrances are 'natural' and which ones are not unless the manufacturer volunteers this information. However, if the product you use does not explicitly state that it includes essential oils, it is probably best to assume that the fragrance portion of the product is synthetic.

Most of us tend to perceive those substances that have a pleasant odour as good and those having an unpleasant odour as harmful. But this is not always the case. Many toxic solvents have a sweetish odour that is not unpleasant, but they can still cause serious harm to health. Each of us has the capability to reduce the number of synthetic fragrances we come into contact with on a daily basis. Choosing the 'fragrance-free' option every time is a simple way to reduce your exposure to lots of complex chemicals that may do more harm than good.

PART TWO

The Products
We Use

It is estimated that each day we expose ourselves to around 200 unique man-made chemicals through our personal-care products alone. Many of these are chemicals that our bodies were never meant to be exposed to, don't metabolise fully and which have been shown, in the lab and in the real world, to cause long-term harm to health.

Avoiding petroleum-derived products not only benefits your health, it makes a positive contribution to saving precious resources as well

The following chapters provide an in-depth look at the sorts of products you use every day, what they contain, what the alternatives are and how you can become more engaged in the process of making healthier choices. What stands out clearly as you begin to dissect the labels of conventional products is why beauty has become more and more of an environmental issue as well as a health issue. Many of the ingredients in our personal-care products rely heavily on a variety of basic ingredients made from petrochemicals. Unless you have been living on the moon or in a cave, you will know that the world is running out of oil and we all need to start thinking differently about all the energy intensive things we do, including our use of toiletries and cosmetics.

In addition to making positive choices like opting for vegetable-based products where available, and brands that are committed to the concept of minimal and recycled packaging, it can be useful to keep the following list of petroleum-derived ingredients in mind when you are in the shops. Avoiding these not only benefits your health, it makes a positive contribution to saving precious resources as well.

Petroleum-derived ingredients

- *Isopropanol* Solvent and penetration enhancer, found in make-up, shampoo, moisturisers and nail polish. Neurotoxic, drying and irritating to skin and potentially liver toxic.
- *Methyl-, Propyl-, Butyl- and Ethyl-Paraben* The most widely used preservatives in the cosmetic industry. Found in most products. Parabens can cause allergic reactions and skin rashes. Studies have shown that they are easily absorbed into the body and once there they have an oestrogenic effect. Oestrogens are known cancer triggers and reproductive toxins, and may be implicated in low sperm counts.
- *Paraffinum Liquidum* Also known as mineral oil (and sometimes listed wrongly as just 'paraffin') it is found in face creams, make-up, body lotions and baby oils, even though it does not add moisture or nourish the skin. Instead, it can interfere with the body's own natural moisturising mechanism, leading to dryness and chapping. It is used because it is cheap and abundant and it gives the false impression that is moisturises.
- *Petrolatum* Also known as petroleum jelly, this mineral-oil derivative is widely used for its emollient properties in cosmetics. Causes similar problems to *paraffinum liquidium*. Found in lipsticks and balms, hair-care products, moisturisers, depilatories and deodorants.
- *Propylene Glycol* Found in moisturisers, deodorants, make-up, depilatories and soaps, it can be derived from natural sources but is usually a synthetic petrochemical mix. It is added to keep the product moist and acts as a penetration enhancer, driving ingredients

deeper into the skin. Can cause allergic reactions, hives and eczema. Ingredients such as *PEG* (*polyethylene glycol*) or *PPG* (*polypropylene glycol*) are related synthetics.

- **PVP/VA Copolymer** A plastic-like substance used in hairspray, styling aids, make-up, fake tan, toothpaste and skin creams. Inhaled particles can damage the lungs of sensitive people.

- **Sodium Lauryl/Laureth Sulfate** Harsh detergents used in shampoos, body washes and toothpaste. Some labels list this ingredient as 'from coconuts'. However, producing *sodium lauryl/laureth sulphate* requires the addition of petroleum-derived ingredients and the finished product is far removed from its vegetable origins. Causes eye irritation, scalp scurf similar to dandruff, skin rashes and allergic reactions.

- **Synthetic Colours** Denoted in Britain and the rest of the EU by the prefix CI followed by several numbers. Most toiletries and cosmetics contain colours even though they add nothing to the effectiveness of the product. Many synthetic colours can be carcinogenic and so are best avoided. Exceptions are mineral-based colours which are denoted with the prefix CI 75- or CI 77-.

- **Parfum** Around 95 per cent of the fragrances used in toiletries and cosmetics are petrochemically based. Often they are made up of dozens of separate ingredients. Perfumes are neurotoxic and can cause headaches, mood swings, depression, dizziness, vomiting and skin irritation. They are also very common triggers of asthma attacks.

- **Toluene** Used as a solvent in cosmetics, especially nail polish and dyes. A toxic, volatile chemical that may irritate the skin and respiratory tract and cause mild anaemia and liver damage with prolonged exposure.

The personal-care industry is one of the most poorly regulated industries in the world. Indeed, because the industry is largely self-regulating it is sometimes a bit of a free-for-all. Over the years its accounting for the health consequences of the ingredients it uses has been very poor, with upwards of 90 per cent of cosmetics ingredients having no relevant safety data at all. Its accounting for its environmental footprint is almost nil.

That means it is up to consumers to ask tougher questions before agreeing to pay for any product. For instance:

- Does the product cause damage to the environment during manufacture, use or disposal?
- Does the product consume a disproportionate amount of energy and other resources during manufacture, use or disposal?
- Does the product cause unnecessary waste, due either to excessive packaging or to a short useful life?
- Does the product use materials derived from threatened species or environments?
- Is the product dangerous to the health of people or animals?
- Does the product involve the unnecessary use of, or cruelty to, animals?

These, of course, are guidelines and it can be difficult to pick a product that is 100 per cent 'good' for you and for the environment. For instance, packaging is a huge and unresolved problem in the personal-care market, even among manufacturers who market themselves as 'green'. For one thing, many products have both primary and secondary packaging. Primary packaging is the bottle or tub or tube it comes in; secondary packaging is the plastic and cardboard stuff around this which makes it look more enticing in the shop. Few manufacturers get it right.

There is also transit packaging, the packaging you never see such as the wooden pallets, board and plastic wrapping and containers that are used to collate products into larger, more manageable loads for transport. In 2001, the UK produced an estimated 9.3 million tonnes of waste packaging. Of this, 5.1 million tonnes came from households and the remaining 4.2 million tonnes from commercial and industrial sources.

In terms of packaging there is a lot of greenwash about *PET* plastic, for example, and how bottles made of this substance can be recycled. In reality recycling any kind of plastic is energy intensive, rarely happens and if it does, only delays the waste process rather than avoiding it. This is because most plastics can only be usefully recycled once. The best thing consumers can do is look for glass packaging that is easily recyclable, and not to buy products with lots of secondary packaging.

It is precisely because this kind of daily policing of what we buy is so hard that it can be preferable to learn to both buy and use less and to be picky about what you do buy.

Chapter 6
Make-up

Many women would argue that make-up is just a bit of fun – a harmless pleasure that makes them feel good about themselves. But the make-up which women put on their faces each day – and wear for long hours at a time – is anything but a benign enhancement of beauty.

There is nothing unique about the ingredients in your favourite make-up. On the whole these will be exactly the same as the ingredients in your face cream and bath and hair products.

By the time a woman has made-up her face she has covered her skin in mineral oil (a carcinogen) and preservatives such as parabens (sensitisers and oestrogen disrupters); *Kathon CG* (a sensitiser, mutagen and suspected carcinogen); and *diazolidinyl urea* (another sensitiser). She will also have exposed herself to synthetic colours, many of which are known carcinogens and allergens; fragrance, the ingredients of which are sensitisers, central nervous system disrupters and carcinogens; plasticisers such as *polyvinylpyrrolidone* (*PVP*), also a carcinogen; surfactants such as *triethanolamine*, film formers such as *dimethicone* and *polytetrafluoroethylene* (*PTFE* or Teflon); talc which is carcinogenic when inhaled and commonly contaminated with heavy metals such as lead and poisons such as arsenic; synthetic waxes derived from petroleum (also potentially carcinogenic); and sunscreens, which are sensitisers and also oestrogen mimics. The list of products you may apply to your face each day is endless – foundation, concealer, powder, blush, mascara, eyeshadow – and the all contain a cocktail of potentially harmful ingredients.

Preservatives

In addition to parabens and *Kathon CG* (the risks of which are detailed in Chapter 2), most types of make-up also contain the preservative *butyl hydroxyanisole (BHA)*, a chemical that is easily absorbed into the skin and which has been designated a human carcinogen by the US National Toxicology Program.

Eye make-up, especially mascaras, can sometimes contain mercury-based preservatives such as *phenylmercuric acetate* and *thimerosal*, the same controversial preservative that is used in some adult vaccines (but has been banned in childhood vaccines because of fears that it can trigger autism and other brain disorders). These are toxic and damaging to the eye. Mercury-based preservatives can also be found in a wide range of toiletries including soap-free cleansers, antiseptic sprays, make-up remover and eye moisturisers.

Thimerosal is not always listed on the label by that name, but instead is called by one of its many synonyms including *mercurochrome, merthiolate, sodium ethylmercurithiosalicylate, thimerosalate, thiomerosalan, merzonin, mertorgan, ethyl (2-mercaptobenzoato-S), mercury sodium salt, merfamin* or *[(o-carboxyphenyl)thi] ethylmercury sodium salt*. A glance at this complicated list and it's easy to see how the use of mercury in a product used on the eyes has escaped the attention of the vast majority of us.

Colours

Most of us try to avoid foods that contain artificial colours. Yet every day women paint their faces with a range of artificial colours known to cause health problems in both the short and long term.

Artificial colours may be carcinogens (indeed, all coal-tar dyes are considered carcinogenic), others may contain hidden carcinogenic impurities in some batches but not in others depending on the source of the raw materials. What's more, cosmetic pigments such as artificial colours can also cause contact dermatitis and irritation.

The problem is that depending on the country of manufacture and the country of sale and depending on how it is used, a colour can be listed on the label by any number of different names. For instance, colours with FD&C prefixes are allowed in foods, drugs and cosmetics; those with a D&C prefix are allowed in drugs and cosmetics only. Many of the same dyes used in cosmetics are also used in foods in the European Union where they are listed as E-numbers. Use the table on p. 23 to help you decipher the label.

Toxic metals

Despite rigorous testing and trials, cosmetics can also contain toxic metals, most commonly as contaminants in pigments and talc. One Finnish study looked at 88 brands of eyeshadow and found that 75 per cent of the products tested contained detectable levels of at least one of the following elements: lead, cobalt, nickel, chromium or arsenic.

In this study the elements found in the cosmetics were impurities in the ingredients rather than listed ingredients – a problem reflected in many cosmetics. While the researchers felt that in most cases these levels were not enough to cause allergic reactions, another study from the UK found that chronic exposures to very low levels of arsenic – lower than those in the Finnish study – were capable of causing hormone disruption.

In 2007, the Campaign for Safe Cosmetics commissioned a series of tests of red lipsticks manufactured in the United States and used daily by millions of women. Twenty of 33 brand-name lipsticks tested contained detectable levels of lead, with levels ranging from 0.03 to 0.65 parts per million (ppm). None of these lipsticks listed lead as an ingredient. To put this in perspective the 'safe' level of lead in confectionary is 0.1ppm.

Lead can harm almost any system in the body but is particularly toxic to the nervous system and while you can be exposed to lead from other sources, for instance air pollution, why would you voluntarily put it on your lips where it is easily swallowed when you lick your lips, eat or drink, as well as being absorbed through the delicate skin and lining of the mouth?

Carcinogens

Liquid formulas such as foundations are subject to the same problems as shampoos and other toiletries (see Chapter 10) in that they often contain the same cancer-causing nitrosamines found in shampoos and foam baths. The longer the product has been on the shelf, the higher the risk of nitrosamine formation. Mascara, especially those types that promise to extend lashes, can also contain carcinogenic plasticisers including *polyurethane*.

Another common ingredient, silica, is usually touted as a natural, skin-enhancing mineral, despite cosmetic silica being synthesised in the lab. In 2000 in the USA, crystalline silica (sometimes called crystalline quartz, and the same ingredient found in cat litter and scouring powders) was added to the National Toxicology Program's list of carcinogens.

While silica can be used in any cosmetic formulation, products such as face powder and eye shadows pose the most risk. The concern here is that the amorphous hydrated form of silica commonly used is cosmetics can be contaminated with carcinogenic crystalline quartz. Unfortunately, it is impossible to tell which silica-containing products are contaminated in this way without undertaking detailed analysis in a laboratory.

A product labelled 'hypoallergenic' may still contain potentially carcinogenic substances

Most make-up, even powder formulas, also contains some form of mineral oil. Mineral oil is the substance that binds powders together and

CONSIDER THIS

Try getting out of the make-up habit. Many women wear make-up for the most trivial occasions, like a trip to the supermarket, picking the kids up from school, weekends at home or walks in the park. Get out of the habit. Get used to the way you look without make-up and give your skin and your system a break. If you can't bear to go out without something on your face, stick to the basics – a swipe of carefully chosen mascara, for instance one made from all natural ingredients, and a bit of lipstick or gloss is fine for everyday wear and has the advantage of lightening your toxic load.

also provides the basis for liquid formulations and lipsticks. Mineral oils were first recognised as carcinogens in 1987. Listed as *parafinnum liquidim* (the stuff that baby oil is made from) or *petrolatum* (petroleum jelly) these highly refined oils have a chequered history. Mineral oils are also thought to increase the photosensitivity of the skin, making it more susceptible to sun-induced damage and skin cancer.

Because the mineral oils used in cosmetics are highly refined, scientists cannot say conclusively how dangerous they are to humans. The thinner the oil, as in *paraffinum liquidum*, the more risky they are thought to be due to the high levels of volatile hydrocarbons thin oils contain. The National Toxicology Program's 9th Report on Carcinogens notes that analyses of mineral oils used for medicinal and cosmetic purposes reveal the presence of several carcinogenic hydrocarbons known as *polycyclic aromatic hydrocarbons*. These include *benzo[b]fluoranthene, benzo[k]fluoranthene* and *benzo[a]pyrene*.

Try this instead

When it comes to make-up, it may be a case of choosing your poison carefully. If the rest of your life is relatively toxin free, the appropriate use of less harmful make-up may not add significantly to your total toxic load. When you do buy or use cosmetics, follow some simple guidelines to help you choose the safest ones.

- **Start on the inside**. Beauty really does come from within. It starts with a nutritious, well-balanced diet, adequate rest and exercise, and periodic breaks from stress. Without these basics, no make-up can make you look beautiful.
- **Read the label**. It is essential to get in to the habit of looking at the ingredients in your cosmetics. Do not rely on claims of 'all natural', 'organic' or 'cruelty free'. These claims are meaningless. The only thing that tells the true story of your cosmetic is the ingredients list. Once you have identified an ingredient or ingredients that you wish to avoid, keep its name on a card or list that you can take with you when you shop. Remember also that price is no guarantee of safety or quality. Sometimes cheaper brands contain fewer toxic ingredients. Only the label will tell you for sure.
- **But don't put too much faith in the label**. Don't just buy a

product because it was safe last time you looked. By the time you are ready to replace your eyeshadow or lipstick it may be made from completely different ingredients. Manufacturers are continually reformulating their products, often according to which ingredients are available and least expensive at the time. In addition many ingredient labels – for instance those used on eyeshadows and lipsticks – list the colours for the entire range rather than the specific product you are buying. For these reasons some products say 'may include' or the symbol '+/-' before a list of ingredients – making it impossible to make sensible choices about safety.

- **Avoid cosmetics that are pearly, glittery, opalescent or frosted**. These are among the most dangerous since to achieve this effect manufacturers add ingredients such as pure aluminium, mica and even fish scales. Used near the eye these particles can flake off and cause corneal damage. Ingested aluminium in particular is linked to Alzheimer's disease. Stick to matt colours, blot well and shine up your lips with a over- or undercoat of shea butter or natural oils.

- **Choose lip gloss** (which has a lower volume of colour ingredients) over lipstick for everyday wear, but be aware, conventional lip glosses contain less colour but can be high in phenol, a poisonous substance that is easily absorbed into the delicate tissue of the lips (aided by the addition of *petrolatum*, a petroleum-derived moisturiser) as well as other wetting agents. Phenol ingestion can cause nausea, vomiting, convulsions, paralysis, respiratory collapse and even death. Minute amounts are linked with skin rashes, swelling, pimples and hives.

- **Seek 'safe' colours**. If you are looking for products with less harmful colours, one easy way to work your way through the maze is remember: in cosmetics a number that begins CI75- is considered a 'natural' colorant, even though some of these are highly synthesised. Anything else may be considered suspect. Those beginning with CI77- are an inorganic substance used as colourings (iron oxides and natural carbon and the more toxic aluminium and barium sulphate fall into this category).

- **Avoid all perfumed cosmetics** and especially avoid those lip products with a sweet taste. Often these include saccharin (a suspected carcinogen) and *phthalic anhydride* (made from another suspected carcinogen, *naphthalene*) is an irritant that can cause headaches, nausea, vomiting, diarrhoea and confusion and has been linked to kidney damage and brain damage in infants. Remarkable then, that it is commonly used in 'play' and 'fun' make-up aimed at young girls.

- **Choose products without sunscreens**. Chances are you are wearing your make-up inside anyway. Also don't be fooled by claims of natural sunscreens. There is no such thing. The only effective sunscreens are synthetic chemicals that add to your toxic load.

How to take off your make-up

The staggering range of different chemicals in your make-up can make taking it off at night a bit of a trial. Cosmetics that are oil-based generally require an oil to dissolve them, which seems preferable to lots of scrubbing with soap and water.

Taking your make-up off at night can become tedious, especially if you are tired, but it is the best thing you can do for your skin, since night-time is when the skin repairs and renews itself. Incorporating a bit of light massage into your facial cleansing routine can also help promote good circulation and enhance the tone and texture of your skin. You don't need expensive cleansers to remove your make-up. What you need can easily be made at home with a few basic ingredients.

- **Use natural oils**. Even if you have oily skin, using a vegetable oil is the best way to get it clean. Simple vegetable oils like sweet almond apricot kernel or grapeseed – or olive or avocado if your skin is very dry or affected by winter weather – can dissolve dirt, oils and make-up residue which have built up on the skin. They will leave your skin feeling very soft. Try applying a warm, damp cloth to your skin first to help loosen dirt and make-up. Apply your chosen oil with clean hands and massage around the face and neck in a circular motion. Wipe off with a flannel, or better still a microfibre cloth. Rinse the cloth and wipe again to remove any remaining traces of grime, rinse with cool water and moisturise as usual.

- **Give yourself a honey facial**. Once a month try using active manuka honey as a cleansing facial. Most honeys can be used as masks for a quick 10-minute skin pick-me-up. Manuka is rich in special enzymes, antioxidants and other nutrients which can have an especially therapeutic and conditioning effect on tired skin.

THE LABEL HYPE

Manufacturers use a variety of terms on product labels to convince us to buy their products. Most of these are meaningless. To make better choices about the products you use, you may find it helpful to know that most of these claims are little more than advertising pitches. Below are some of the most common claims that you wil find on make-up and beauty products, and what they really mean.

Hypoallergenic

Many products now claim to be hypoallergenic. 'Hypo' means 'sub' or 'below' and the true meaning of the word 'hypoallergenic' is not 'allergen free' but 'lower in known allergens'. There are no regulations defining what an allergen is, though years of consumer complaint and dissatisfaction has defined many of the most common skin allergens in cosmetics, toiletries and household products. Equally, there are no official guidelines for producing hypoallergenic products. What is more, a product which is hypoallergenic may still contain substances which may be potentially carcinogenic or harmful to human health in some other way.

Fragrance-free

Many of us will buy a fragrance-free product because we experience an allergic reaction to fragrance or because we are seeking to cut down on the amount of perfumes we use on a daily basis. But even fragrance-free products can have a recognisable scent. This is because while many fragrance-free products do not contain perfumes they can contain the raw ingredients of fragrance, often included to mask the odour of other chemicals.

In reality, going fragrance-free is also only half the battle for sensitive individuals. While most fragrance-free products are free of colour this is not always the case. Cosmetic colours are also a significant source of allergic reactions such as dermatitis.

pH balanced

pH is measured on a scale of 0 (highly acid) to 14 (highly alkali), with 7 being considered neutral. 'Normal' skin pH ranges from 5–8. Contrary to what you have heard, the skin and hair do not have an official pH, though generally the skin is more acid than alkali. Skin produces keratin, fatty acids and other substances that work continuously to adjust its pH level. Almost anything you put on your skin, including water, will temporarily alter its pH. The pH of your skin can also change according to your environment and your state of health.

In reality there is no such thing as a pH-balanced product anyway. The product that left the factory with one pH may shift substantially during storage and shift again when applied to your hair or body and according to the pH of the water it is being used in. Unless it is very harsh and applied continuously, the pH of a product will not alter the pH of the skin substantially or for long.

Clinically proven

A claim of clinically proven is an effective sales pitch. Companies that make a claim like that should have competent and reliable scientific evidence to back it up, in most cases with well-controlled clinical studies. Their products should be tested on humans, not on animals or in the test tube, but this is not always the case. Because there is no legal definition of what clinically proven means, it can mean virtually anything, including nothing.

Dermatologist tested

Similar to clinically proven, this claim implies a product was tested by a dermatologist and shown to not cause any skin reactions. While it may sound reassuring, manufacturers are not required to perform any tests or provide supporting evidence to demonstrate that products labelled 'dermatologist-tested' were actually tested by a doctor and produced fewer allergic reactions than other products.

Chapter 7

Skin Care – Your Body

Body lotions, creams and gels are an integral part of many women's beauty routine. The ingredients of a typical body lotion are not much different from those of a hair conditioner. And the two products basically perform the same function – replacing natural oils with synthetic ones and then coating the skin with a thin waterproof layer.

While most moisturisers promise miraculous effects, several of the ingredients commonly used in body lotions can make the skin drier and more permeable, allowing other toxic ingredients to be absorbed into the body. There is also some evidence that moisturisers can make the skin more susceptible to damage caused by synthetic detergents used in many facial and body care products.

You may think that body oil seems like a more straightforward alternative to complicated cream or lotion mixtures, yet many are based on mineral oil. Some, like baby oil, are 100 per cent mineral oil (*paraffinum liquidum*) with added perfume.

Mineral oil, a by-product of the distillation of gasoline from crude oil, impedes the skin's ability to breathe, attract moisture and detoxify. It can also slow down cell renewal and promote premature skin ageing. It is used for its lubricant qualities which in the short term appear to make the skin softer, used over the longer term, however, mineral oil can make the skin dry out. This is because mineral oil dissolves the skin's natural oils, thereby increasing water-loss from the skin.

Any mineral oil derivative can be contaminated with cancer-causing *polycyclic aromatic hydrocarbons* (*PAHs*). Mineral oils may also increase the skin's sensitivity to sunlight and have been linked to an increased risk of skin cancer. *Petrolatum*, paraffin or paraffin oil and *propylene glycol* are all forms of mineral oil.

Among women who switch toiletry brands or try new products, mineral oils have been shown to be the major cause of new skin irritation, including rashes and spots. There is no good reason for this kind of suffering. Given the risks associated with mineral oils, some manufacturers have switched to using silicone-based oils and gels.

Silicones such as *dimethicone* (or *dimethiconol*), *cyclomethicone*, *cyclopentasiloxane* and *cyclohexasiloxane* are synthesised from silicon metal to produce water repellent 'dry' oils and waxes. They provide many of the feel-good qualities associated with modern body-care products such as texture, silkiness, lustre and smooth application.

Silicones come in many forms. Film-forming silicones add spreadability and smoothness as well as water repellence to products such as facial cosmetics, lotions, creams, antiperspirants and deodorants. In cosmetics like lipsticks, eye shadows and blushers, silicone resins and gums provide longevity to help the product to stay on the skin and maintain its colour and they improve control in hair styling products. When used as surfactants and conditioners in hair products, silicones add foam stabilisation to add shine, body and softness to the hair. Volatile silicones evaporate quickly. They make aesthetically pleasing and effective anti-perspirants and deodorants that do not leave a residue. Highly reflective silicones enhance the shine of surfaces such as skin and hair. Silicones are also widely used in household cleaning products, including laundry detergents, fabric softeners, polishes and waxes.

On the whole, silicones allow the skin to breathe better than mineral oils, but their long-term safety is by no means guaranteed. While they increase the feel-good factor of a product, they are poorly absorbed by the skin and this places a question mark over how well ingredients suspended in them will be absorbed. Some like, *dimethicone*, are also cancer suspects.

- **Use natural oils**. Effective moisturisers can be prepared on an 'as needed' basis by everyone from a simple mixture of vegetable or biological oils (coconut, jojoba, almond or emu) and plant 'butters' (shea or mango), water and glycerine. With practice these can be made to suit different areas of the body and respond to the skin's seasonal needs (i.e. heavier oils in winter, lighter ones in summer).

  The advantage of natural oils is that they contain all the nutrients natural to the plant or animal. Many such as jojoba and emu are amazingly similar to the oils in human skin and as such are non-irritating, don't clog pores and are deeply nourishing.

  If you are going to continue to use commercial products, choose those with the fewest ingredients and watch out in particular for those that may be contaminated with carcinogens. It is the oil and wax content of moisturisers that holds moisture next to the skin, so why not consider simple vegetable oils to maintain the skin's suppleness. They will do the same job at a fraction of the price and you'll have the advantage of actually knowing what you are putting on your body

  As a general rule, use lighter oils such as apricot kernel, coconut or jojoba oil for normal skins and heavier oils such as avocado and evening primrose oil for older or drier skins. Rosehip oil is considered a rich and nourishing oil for the face.

- **For dry skin**. If your skin is occasionally dry consider using natural oils after bathing or washing to temporarily seal in moisture. See Chapter 9 for tips on using oils in the bath.

Hand and nail creams

Like body oils and lotions, hand and nail creams are essentially mineral oil based. There is little difference between the ingredients of most body lotions and those which are supposed to be specifically for the hands, although hand creams tend to have even more emollients in them. Hands become dry and cracked because they are more exposed to the elements and more in use than almost any other part of the body. You also wash your hands more often and expose them to detergents and other cleaning products more often as well.

While not as thin as facial skin, the skin on your hands is still thin enough to allow the penetration of noxious chemicals. To keep them soft, and to avoid absorbing toxic chemicals into your body, always use gloves when doing cleaning jobs, and substitute vegetable oils and vegetable oil-based creams for petroleum-based ones.

The condition of your nails and cuticles depends on a healthy varied diet rich in vitamins and minerals. The sorts of harsh chemicals we come into contact with on a daily basis – for instance chlorine from swimming pools, cleaning products, nail enamel and acetone-based polish removers – can wreak havoc on your nails, making them brittle and causing the skin around them to become dry and ragged.

Try the simple maintenance routine of rubbing the contents of a Vitamin E capsule or a touch of wheatgerm oil into the nails and cuticles to help improve nail condition and prevent them drying out. If your nails are very dirty, for instance if you have been working with paints or in the garden, try digging your fingernails into lemon halves then scrub vigorously with a brush dipped in apple cider vinegar.

Rub the contents of a Vitamin E capsule on your nails to prevent them drying out

Nails are made up largely of a keratin protein and a combination of minerals including calcium, sulphur, potassium and selenium. You can help build healthy nails from the inside out by including more proteins and minerals in your diet. Spirulina, a blue-green micro algae from the sea, is a source of easily digestible protein. It also contains minerals, beta-carotene and fatty acids.

Your nails may reflect the health of your liver. If your nails are weak or misshapen then it could mean your liver needs a boost. Try avoiding alcohol for a while; adopt a low-fat diet drinking plenty of fresh vegetable juices – especially beetroot, carrot, cucumber and apple.

Foot creams

When your feet are tired, it seems the whole of your body feels tired. Feet take a lot of strain each day and whilst rubbing them with cream can be soothing and keeps them soft, the best way to take care of your feet it to put them up from time to time and to walk barefoot as much as possible. What makes feet tired and gives them corns, bunions and rough skin is not just standing but squeezing them into often poorly fitting shoes and impossibly high heels.

Conventional foot creams contain many of the same ingredients as other body creams, though tend to be more concentrated to penetrate the thicker and sometimes drier skin on the soles of the foot.

Well fitting and supportive shoes, good posture (almost impossible to maintain, by the way, in high heels), soaking your feet in a soothing footbath, resting with them elevated from time to time and massaging them with an aromatherapy oil will make a huge difference to your wellbeing from the ground up.

Consider these foot-care alternatives:

- **Give your feet a massage**. Do this by going to a professional reflexologist, which can be very rewarding and have other health benefits too. The nerves and channels (or 'reflex points') in the feet are a way to stimulate other parts of the body such as your internal organs. But you don't have to be a professional or go to one to get these benefits. Make a simple oil mixture of 75ml (5tbsp) of light oil such as almond or apricot kernel oil and mix 20 drops of an essential oil of your choice (peppermint, bergamot, mandarin, lavender, thyme and patchouli are all suitable). You can use this to give each foot an invigorating 10-minute massage, paying special attention to any places that feel sore or tender. Put a pair of socks on and put your feet up for a few minutes once you have finished.

- **Make a foot scrub**. Mix a little salt with almost any base oil (olive and grapeseed are good) and you can use this to work on the dry skin areas of your feet. For really tough or thick areas of dry skin, soak your feet for 10 minutes then use a natural pumice stone to remove dry flaky skin.

- **Try a footbath**. If you are very tired and your feet are very sore, try soaking your feet in a warm, shallow bath (a simple plastic basin will do) of Epsom salts. Just add a handful to the water and stir it up to make sure they dissolved. Alternatively, you can make a more luxurious footbath with warm water and a mixture of essential oils such as lavender, patchouli and sandalwood. To disperse the oils evenly in the water add a splash of milk and mix well. If you suffer from itchy feet or athlete's foot, try adding 125ml (4floz) of vinegar to a tepid footbath. For an easy invigorating foot massage put some pebbles into a shallow basin, cover with cold water and run your feet over these slowly and firmly for 10 minutes.

- **Use footsocks**. They may not be sexy but applying a good quality oil or natural moisturiser to your feet after you bathe, and then popping on a pair of trainer socks will help keep feet moisturised. Do this once a week as a treat for your feet.

Sun creams

Sun exposure and the use of sunblocks and sunscreens is one of the most complex and contradictory areas of skin health. On the one hand, exposure to the fresh air and sun is vital for a healthy body. Sunlight is an important source of Vitamin D necessary for development and the maintenance of bones and teeth. But at the same time, too much sun exposure can raise your risk of skin cancer.

Relying on sunscreens as your sole means of protection is fraught with problems since the protection they offer is never guaranteed. Furthermore, most commercial sun creams contain a mixture of harsh and harmful chemicals that present their own risks. For example, some of the chemicals in sunscreens are thought to cause disruption or permanent damage to the nervous, immune and respiratory systems. Young children may be especially susceptible to sunscreen chemicals and their toxic-side effects. Among the most harmful are *benzophenones*, which can cause allergic reactions, and *PABA*s which have been shown to form carcinogenic *nitrosamines* when mixed with other chemicals.

The effectiveness of any sun cream depends on its UV absorption, its concentration, formulation and ability to withstand swimming or sweating. As a general rule, the higher the sun protection factor (SPF) the greater the number of chemicals in a sun lotion or cream. It is not uncommon for sun creams to contain three or more sunscreen agents as well as perfumes, insect repellents and a host of other chemicals besides. Though many of the ingredients used in sunscreens have been tested individually, studies of the long-term effects of combinations of sunscreen agents, applied liberally over an extended period of time are rare.

There are two main types of ultraviolet rays, UVA and UVB. The SPF factor in your sun cream is for protection against UVB rays only, most of which are filtered out by the ozone layer. Those that do get through stimulate the skin's pigment to produce melanin, our natural defence against sunlight. UVA rays are not filtered out by the ozone layer and penetrate the skin at a deeper level, so they have the potential to cause more skin damage. Gauging UVA protection is a little more difficult, though most creams now put UVA information on their labels as well.

Some experts believe that, when exposed to UV rays, sunscreens like *oxybenzone* can break down into chemicals that destroy or inhibit the skin's natural defences against sunlight. This leaves it vulnerable to the free radicals produced by exposure to sunlight. Free radicals are the toxic by-products of metabolism. Free-radical damage to the skin is implicated in skin cancer, premature ageing and other damage to the skin.

Similarly, sunscreens such as *padimate-O* are thought to absorb harmful UV rays. But as scientists point out, once absorbed this energy still has to be released somewhere, usually directly onto the skin where it is metabolised into free radicals which can actually increase the risk of skin cancer.

What's in your sun cream?

There are two basic types of creams available on the market today: chemical sunscreens, which act by absorbing ultraviolet light, and chemical sunblocks, which reflect or scatter light in both the visible and UV spectrum. Both types are associated with skin irritation.

These are the most common chemical sunscreens:

- **Benzophenones** are common skin sensitisers and can provoke allergic reactions in some individuals. Common *benzophenones* include *oxybenzone, dioxybenzone* and *sulisbenzone*.
- **PABAs** are formaldehyde-forming chemicals that can form carcinogenic *nitrosamines* when combined with amines such as *DEA, TEA* and *MEA* in the mixture. *PABAs* can cause skin irritation. Common *PABAs* are *p-aminobenzoic acid, ethyl dihydroxypropyl PABA, padimate-O (ocyl dimethyl PABA), padimate A* and *glyceryl PABA*.
- **Cinnamates** are common skin irritants. This group of chemicals includes *cinoxate, ethylhexyl-p-methoxycinnamate, octocrylene* and *ocytl methoxycinnamate*.
- **Salicylates** are also skin irritants and are associated with a high rate of

dermatitis among users. Those commonly used in sun creams include *ethylhexyl salicylate, homosalate, octyl salicylate* and *neo-homosalate.*

- Other common sunscreen agents include *methyl anthranilate, digalloyl trioleate* and *avobenzone (butyl methoxy-dibenzoylmethane).*
- The most commonly used chemical **sunblocks** are: *zinc oxide, titanium dioxide* and *red petrolatum.*
- Bear in mind that in addition to sunscreens, sun creams also inevitably include all the same ingredients as body lotions such as mineral and other synthetic oils, *PEGs, TEA* and other surfactants, preservatives and fragrances.

Faking it

There are two ways to get a tan without exposure to the sun: using a sunbed or applying fake tan.

Sunbeds produce ultraviolet rays, just like the sun. In fact, a sunbed can be even more dangerous than the sun. It's estimated that 20 minutes in a solarium can be equivalent to approximately four hours in the sun.

Sunlight contains a mix of UVA and UVB radiation and some of this is filtered out by the ozone layer. Sunbeds produce mainly UVA radiation, which penetrates deeper into your skin. They produce less UVB radiation than the sun.

People using sunbeds are less likely to use sun cream to protect themselves against UV radiation. Goggles are essential – as with sunshine, the combination of UVA and UVB can result in eye damage by burning the cornea. Long-term exposure can result in irreversible damage and cataracts. Sunbeds can also accelerate the thinning of the skin, the development of wrinkles and fine lines, and other changes usually associated with ageing.

In the 1950s, the first self-tanning product came on the market. There are now hundreds of cosmetics products marketed as a safe and effective alternative to direct sun exposure. But while products like these are widely promoted as a safe alternative to sun exposure, there are, inevitably, problems.

First of all, self-tanning lotions offer little protection from UV radiation. So if you're taking a trip outside in the sunshine to show off your new fake tan, you'll still need to use some suncream. Next, it's worth considering how self-tanning products work to colour your skin.

The most effective products contain a chemical called *dihydroxyacetone* (*DHA*). This sugar derivative has been the staple active ingredient in self-tanners for many years. It can smell bad and it can sometimes turn you a strange shade of orange, but more importantly, it has never been fully evaluated for safety. *DHA* is not a dye. It imparts temporary colour to the skin through a free-radical-generating chemical reaction with the amino acids in superficial layers of the skin. The way it works is not dissimilar to the way exposure to the air can turn a cut-up apple brown.

Some products also use another chemical, *erythrulose*, in addition to the *DHA*. *Erythrulose* works identically to *DHA*, but develops more slowly. The two chemicals used together may produce a longer-lasting effect.

Both *dihydroxyacetone* and *erythrulose* may cause contact dermatitis, but there is a greater irony here that won't be lost on those who have ever skimmed a women's magazine. Most anti-ageing creams, for instance, include ingredients that help fight the damaging, skin-ageing effects of free radicals, which are known to promote premature skin cell death. Using a fake tan means volunteering for this kind of damage to your skin, and a 2004 study underscored this fact with the finding that *DHA* interferes with the normal cell cycle in human skin, induces DNA damage, and accelerates cell death within 24 hours of application. This alarming study was one of only a very few attempts to explore how safe fake tan promoters are; *erythrulose*, for example, has never been fully evaluated for long-term safety.

Fake tan products also suffer from the same plethora of toxic ingredients as body lotions. Often they include numerous film formers; not just silicones but also the plasticiser *tri-C14-15 alkyl citrate* (which is just as frequently found in food packaging). These make application easier but a side effect is that it acts like plastic wrap on the skin, keeping it from eliminating toxins.

Try this instead

Recent research in the *British Medical Journal* suggests that individuals who use sunscreens may actually be at an increased risk of developing skin cancer. This is because high SPF creams give sun worshippers a false sense of security, encouraging them to venture outside during peak

NATURAL SUNSCREENS?

Read labels for natural and 'organic' sunscreens carefully. Usually they are simply the same old ingredients with added plant extracts and oils. Can the addition of these natural ingredients really prevent against sunburn? No, of course not:

- **Aqua** – water does not prevent sunburn.
- **Glycerin** – a lubricant used in moisturizers to make them feel good and go on more smoothly. It has no sun-blocking ability but can dry the skin, making it more vulnerable to sun damage.
- **Octyl palmitate** – a relative of vitamin C. There is no evidence that it can provide protection from the sun.
- **Retinyl palmitate** – also known as pro-Vitamin A or pro-retinol. There is no evidence of sun protection.
- **Tocopherol acetate** – a relative of Vitamin E. Again, there is no evidence it has any effect as a sunscreen.

Other natural ingredients including aloe vera, carrot oil, chamomile, borage oil and avocado oil are used as fillers, stabilizers or preservatives. They are seldom present in high enough quantities to protect or nourish your skin, and none of them have proven sun-blocking ability.

The latest controversy in natural sunscreens concerns microfine particles of zinc oxide and titanium dioxide. These are of course effective sunblocks that have been used for years. But they tend to leave a whitish sheen on the skin and so manufacturers have turned to nanotechnology to try and solve the problem. Most sunblocks on the market now make use of nanoparticles of zinc oxide and titanium dioxide that in theory are small enough to slip through the upper layers of the skin. While manufacturers say these particles are perfectly safe, no study has yet been done to find out how much more the body absorbs of these nanoscale particles and what the potential health effects might be.

In 2006 a US laboratory study found that nanoscale titanium oxide could upset the chemical balance of the brain and produce brain damage. Such results add to a growing body of evidence that suggests that the safety of nanoscale ingredients cannot be taken for granted simply because larger particles of the same substance have no ill effects.

periods and to stay out in the sun much longer than would normally be considered safe.

It is also because of the mix of ingredients in sun cream and the damaging effects they have on the skin. The only safe recommendation is not to rely on sunscreens as your sole method of protection – long sleeves, a hat and staying in the shade are easy ways to keep safe. There is no doubt that sunscreens can be useful, but they should not be applied to large areas of the body over an extended period of time.

Around 80 per cent of our total lifetime exposure to the sun comes during childhood. So it is especially important to make sure children have some protection from strong sunlight. If you want to teach your children good sun-exposure habits, lead by example. Research into children's voluntary use of sun creams, for example, suggests that they copy what their parents do. Consider these simple strategies for enjoying the sun safely:

- **Limit your exposure**. If you want a glow that is truly healthy then regular moderate sun exposure is the only way to go. This does not mean foolishly baking in the sun for hours but rather enjoying the sun as a natural part of your daily routine. Studies show that we all need approximately 15–20 minutes of sun exposure on our face, arms and legs each day to produce and maintain vital supplies of Vitamin D. Staying out of the sun means many of us do not get enough Vitamin D and this has led to the re-emergence of diseases like rickets and contributed to spiralling rates of depression as well as cancers of the breast, prostate and colon.
- **Keep babies under 6 months old out of strong sunlight**. Baby sun creams with a high SPF probably have the greatest number of toxic chemicals and are not suitable for the delicate and permeable skin of babies.
- **Limit time in the sun**. It is probably best to avoid being out when the sun is at its strongest, between the hours of 11am and 2pm.
- **Cover up**. When you and your children are going to be out in the sun for extended periods of time, make practical use of T-shirts, sunglasses, hats and beach umbrellas.
- **If you do get sunburned**, aloe vera gel is soothing and helps repair skin. A cool bath to which you have added either apple cider vinegar

or bicarbonate of soda can help reduce swelling and pain. Use the oat-based wash bag (see p. 89) as a water conditioner for your bath. Make up as directed then leave a bag to steep in a tepid bath. Squeeze it from time to time to release a soothing milk that will help condition your skin while you soak. Freeze wet herbal tea bags (chamomile, nettle and sage are good choices) and apply them for on-the-spot relief.

Chapter 8

Skin Care – Your Face

The amount of stuff we put on our faces is simply staggering, and since facial skin is thinner than skin elsewhere, the potential for absorbing toxic chemicals is much greater. While most skin-care products promise to help us look younger, prolonged use can dry and age the skin considerably. It may not show when you start using them in your 20s but by the time you are in your 50s the damage will be noticeable and mostly irreversible.

- **Cleansing lotions** are often touted as a better way to clean make-up and grime from your face than using plain soap. Lotions and creams, we are told, can clean without stripping away the skin's natural oils (although products containing solvents will dissolve natural oils, usually replacing them with synthetic ones). The ingredients of most cleansing lotions are nearly indistinguishable from those of facial moisturisers. Furthermore, even the simplest cleansing lotion can contain a range of suspect chemicals.
- **Liquid face washes** are similar in their content to liquid body washes (see p. 90) but contain slightly more water. Because liquids are more complex to make than solids, they generally contain more potentially harmful chemicals than detergent bars.

- **Exfoliating scrubs** typically contain harsh detergents, emulsifiers and abrasives. An abrasive can be anything from ground fruit pips to talc, to more worrying particles such as aluminium oxide. Others contain skin-drying agents such as alcohol. A simple flannel will do the job just as well so it is a bit silly to invest in anything else. Exfoliants are a waste of money, may unnecessarily damage your skin through over-enthusiastic use, and will certainly add to your body's toxic load.
- **Moisturisers** are a basic part of many women's – and these days men's – daily routine. As detailed in Chapter 4, moisturisers contain a mixture of often synthetic fats and waxes as well as film formers such as silicones and Teflon. Their purpose is to keep the superficial layers of the skin hydrated and to make it feel temporarily smoother. Facial moisturisers tend to be a bit lighter to wear than those for the body but are basically composed of the same ingredients.
- **Toners** are now accepted as the necessary intermediate step between cleansing and moisturising. In fact this step is an invention of the marketing world. Clean skin is probably as toned as it needs to be.

Many toners use alcohol to dry the skin and make it feel tighter. Others promise to close your pores thus making skin look younger and firmer. Unfortunately, your pore size is genetically determined and pores do not open and close. If they did your face would wobble like a jelly throughout the day. What toner does is put astringent chemicals on you face that lower the skin temperature. This affects the underlying tissue that will temporarily contract giving that characteristic 'tight' feeling which you get after using a toner.

The life of skin

Skin has a life of its own that most of us never hear about. Getting in touch with its natural rhythm, rather than bullying it into submission with lots of creams and potions, is the most straightforward path to a better complexion.

Flip through any magazine or browse in any shop and you will be confronted with a bewildering array of products that promise great skin all day every day. But perfect unchanging skin is only the preserve of celebrities and models who inhabit a world of perpetually good lighting, professional make-up artists and Photoshop.

In reality, skin is a mirror, reflecting and reacting to what you eat and drink, your exposure to environmental pollutants, allergens, cosmetic irritants and the elements. How well you sleep and the stresses you are under are also relevant to the way your skin looks from day to day.

In real people it is in the nature of healthy, normal skin to change on almost an hourly basis. Studies show, for instance, that:

- Production of new skin cells is highest at midnight and lowest at noon.
- Oil production in the skin is twice as high at noon than it is at 2am
- Your skin is more likely to absorb what you put onto it at 4pm than at 8am.
- You're more likely to have an allergic skin reaction in the morning than later in the day.

Normal skin changes are not problems that need to be fixed and there's no getting round the fact that if you want great skin there are no shortcuts and no miracle products. Acknowledging this means you can stop obsessing over the most minute and transient shifts in skin tone and colour, and adopt a more sensible approach to skin care that works from the inside out.

Adjusting your lifestyle to include sleeping longer, eating better, drinking more water and varying your exercise routine can help

SHAVING CREAM

Wet shaving with a blade is one of the oldest ways of removing unwanted hair (from any part of the body). There are now a wide variety of shaving creams, foams and gels on the market for both men and women. They look nice, they feel nice and some even smell nice. But they can contain some not-so-nice ingredients, for example *triethanolamine (TEA)* and *lauramide DEA, PEG-150 distearate, BHT* and *imidazolidinyl urea, parabens, quaternium 15, paraffinum liquidum* and propellants such as *isobutane* and *propane*.

mitigate some of the natural changes that take place at skin level. Ultimately, accepting and working with these may make the difference between being at war, or making peace, with the way you look.

Despite the fact that good skin begins on the inside, the skin-care market is overflowing with choices, which promise to keep you young and wrinkle-free while removing dirt, oil and make-up.

TRY THIS INSTEAD

A wet shave should be a wet shave. Getting hair thoroughly wet before shaving means you can use less cream or foam to get the job done. Modern shaving creams are loaded with lubricants because most men and women skip the essential wetting part of the shave. In addition:

- **Use a shaving soap.** It won't be a soap really (unless you buy it at a specialist natural healthcare shop), but a detergent bar. However, you will be able to avoid the problems associated with solvents and propellants found in shaving foams. Use a brush to get lots of foam unless you have very dry skin as a shaving brush may irritate dry skin. If this is the case, soap up on your hands first before applying the foam to your skin.
- **Use shaving oil.** More and more companies are making nice shaving oils that usually contain added essential oils to smooth and soothe the surface of the face while shaving. Opt for vegetable oil bases in favour of mineral oils.
- **Make your own shaving oil.** In a base of 40ml (2½ tbsp) apricot kernel oil mix the following ingredients 40ml (2½ tbsp) Castile soap, 6 drops bergamot essential oil, 4 drops cedarwood essential oil. Pour the mixture into a bottle and shake well before use. Apply to warm damp skin before shaving.
- **Buy an electric shaver.** The shave won't usually be so close, but it avoids a lot of unnecessary exposure to harsh chemicals.

A closer look at wrinkles

How skin ages is a complicated process involving a number of internal and external factors, some of which are within our control, many of which are not.

Ageing causes decreases in collagen and elastin, the 'scaffolding' of the skin, causing the skin to wrinkle and sag. Gravity can also make loose skin around eyes and jowls sag even more. Aged skin also appears more translucent because of the decrease in the number of pigment-containing cells (melanocytes). It is also thinner and more fragile, and at increased risk of injury and less able to repair itself. Your genetic inheritance is also influential, as are hormonal changes at menopause, though human studies have failed to conclusively link oestrogen decline with skin wrinkles.

An unhealthy lifestyle will be reflected in your skin's condition. Prematurely ageing skin often mirrors the body's inefficiency in eliminating toxins and waste products. Addressing the source of the problem, for instance through diet (see box, p. 80), rather than simply relying on topical creams and lotions, is always preferable.

It has long been believed that sun exposure is the single external biggest cause of wrinkles. But is this true? Excess sun exposure can generate skin-damaging free radicals, leading to what scientists call 'photoageing' (rather than chronological ageing). UVA exposure is believed to be particularly harmful since it leads to the breakdown of the skin's collagen fibres.

But it can be difficult to differentiate between genetically normal wrinkles and those caused by the sun. In addition, a recent study challenged received wisdom by suggesting that people with very wrinkled faces were 90 per cent less likely to get basal-cell carcinoma (BCC), the most common form of skin cancer, even though they had the same amount of sun exposure as cancer victims.

The key difference is the way that older, smooth skin repairs itself – by stimulating the production of transforming growth factor-beta (TGF-) which in turn suppresses the immune system and promotes blood vessel growth – both risk factors for cancer. If confirmed this would quash the broadly accepted idea that wrinkling is an indicator of sunlight-induced damage and therefore of skin cancer risk.

Smoking increases the breakdown of collagen as well as drying the skin and reducing circulation – thus depriving the skin of oxygen and essential nutrients. Smoking may also lower levels of skin-protective Vitamin A. Research shows that smoking 20 cigarettes per day over just a few years is equivalent to almost 10 years of chronological ageing – a much greater rate of damage than lifelong sun exposure.

Do anti-wrinkle creams cause wrinkles?

Many people who scan food labels for harmful additives unthinkingly use toiletries containing a multitude of undesirable chemicals, believing that what we put on our bodies is not as influential to health as what we put in them.

Yet facial skin is thinner than skin elsewhere, and may absorb toxic chemicals (such as petroleum by-products, carcinogens such as *nitrosamines* and *formaldehyde*, solvents and oestrogenic preservatives such as *parabens*) at a much greater rate.

Some sun creams are blamed for making us more vulnerable to skin cancer

Recent attitudes to sun exposure means it can be very difficult to find a commercial moisturiser without a sunscreen. Even some night creams now contain sunscreening agents! Increasingly, sun creams are blamed for making us vulnerable to skin cancer. What is more, if you work outdoors you will probably need more protection than a moisturising cream can give, and if you work in an office all day an added sunscreen is just another unnecessary chemical. So you can very easily reduce the number of chemicals you put on your face each day by using a moisturiser that does not contain an SPF, and only using sunscreens when necessary.

In order to look younger many women remove the superficial layers of skin with harsh exfoliants and chemical peels such as *alpha-hydroxy acids*, *glycolic*, *hydroxycaprylic* or lactic acid, passionflower or citrus extract. Widely believed to improve sun-damaged skin, offer UV protection and heal sunburn damage, recent evidence suggests that these ingredients actually cause premature ageing as well as increased UV susceptibility.

SKIN FOOD

Diet can significantly affect the skin and its tendency to wrinkle. Australian researchers studied the diets of 453 people aged 70 years and over from Australia, Greece and Sweden to find out if particular foods either predicted or were associated with skin wrinkling. The findings strongly suggest that a high intake of fruits, vegetables and fish, as well as certain healthy fats, can reduce skin wrinkling.

Foods that protect against wrinkles
- Higher total fat
- Mono-unsaturated fat (especially avocado and peanut butter)
- Olive oil and olives
- Fish (especially fatty fish)
- Reduced-fat milk and milk products
- Eggs
- Nuts, beans and pulses (especially lima and broad beans)
- Vegetables (especially leafy greens, spinach, aubergine, asparagus, celery, onions, leeks and garlic)
- Wholegrain cereals
- Fruit and fruit products (especially prunes, cherries, apples and jams)
- Tea (preferably without milk, as the addition of milk reduces tea's antioxidant properties)
- Water
- Zinc-containing foods (seafood, lean meat, milk and nuts)

Foods that promote wrinkles
- Saturated fat
- Meat (especially fatty processed meats)
- Full-fat dairy products (especially unfermented products and ice cream)
- Soft drinks and cordials
- Cakes, pastries and desserts
- Potatoes
- Butter
- Margarine

Better alternatives

The most important factor in a face cream is its ability to moisturise. Today, mineral oils (*paraffinum liquidum, petrolatum*) have been largely abandoned in favour of semi-synthetic lipids (fats and oils) and their constituents including *ceramide, hyaluronic acid,* cholesterol, *triglycerides, phospholipids* and glycerine. Synthetic humecants (ingredients which draw water to the skin) include *propylene glycol* and glycerine (which can be animal or vegetable in origin). Many also include silicones (*dimethicone* and various *siloxanes*).

> *The simpler your facial care routine, the better it will be for your face*

Even among the so-called natural alternatives, there are very few products with documented scientific evidence of benefits. Most claims are based on animal studies and the 'science' of guesswork.

Added antioxidants may be helpful to the skin. A handful of studies for instance, suggest that *coenzyme-Q10* (*ubiquinone*) smoothes wrinkles. Vitamin E, either as *alpha tocopherol* or as *tocotrienols*, is an antioxidant which when added to a cream can help prolong the product's shelf life. Some studies suggest it can also smooth superficial wrinkles if used continuously.

Vitamins C and E probably work best against sun damage in combination. Vitamin E can also work synergistically with *carotenoids* (such as *beta carotene* and *retinal*). *Alpha lipoic acid* (*ALA*) scavenges both water and fat-soluble free radicals, sparing levels of Vitamin C and E in the skin. *ALA* is rapidly available to skin cells and may also have some UV protecting properties. Many plant extracts, including those from cocoa and green tea, as well as rosehip oil and horsetail, are also antioxidant.

In reality, you don't need a raft of specialist products to clean or moisturise your face. The simpler your facial-care routine is, the better it will be for your face. Try incorporating the following advice into your daily routine:

- Try to **avoid liquid cleansers**, which are more expensive and have more harsh chemicals in them than solid version. If you want to use conventional bars, **opt for glycerine-based soaps**, which are among the mildest.

- **Switch from detergent bars to castile or pure vegetable oil soaps.** These will clean your face without stripping it completely of natural, beneficial and protective oils (and you won't need to invest in separate bars for body and face).

- Whatever you use, remember to **rinse well.** Residues left behind by neglectful rinsing can irritate skin.

- You can **tone your face simply and easily by splashing on cold water.** The main purpose of a toner is to remove the last bits of cleanser and/or grime and to stimulate circulation and hydrate and refine the skin surface. If you absolutely need to buy something to 'tone' your skin, buy simple products like distilled witch hazel or try using a weak solution of cider vinegar in demineralised water. Aloe vera juice is also a good choice for all skin types because of its astringent, antiseptic and healing properties. Likewise, you can dilute 5ml (1tsp) of white vinegar in 70ml (5tbsp) of purified water to make a toner that is cleansing, invigorating and that helps to restore the skin's pH balance after cleansing.

- **Make a facial scrub.** Avoid using harsh scrubs on your face – and this includes the kinds of salt and sugar scrubs recommended in the body-care section. Instead, opt for softer scrubs made from grains and seeds. These should be ground very finely in a pestle and mortar or in a coffee grinder. Good choices include oatmeal, rice flour, fine clays like bentonite or Fuller's earth. Put 30ml (2tbsp) of any of these (or make a mixture of grains and clay) in a bowl with enough water (or you can use honey, yogurt, milk or even olive oil) to make a paste. Spread the paste on your damp face in a gentle circular motion. Rinse with plenty of water and remove any excess with a soft cloth.

- **Make a facial mask.** Most skin types can benefit from a mask treatment once every couple of weeks. There are two types of facial masks: wet and dry. A wet mask is good for older skin and can help hydrate and soothe. You can make simple wet masks by mixing 30ml (2tbsp) manuka honey and 5ml (1sp) oil (for instance avocado for drier skin or apricot kernel oil for oilier skin; see p.93 for suggestions), or alternatively mix with a plant gel like aloe, or a little rosewater. Leave on for 10 minutes and rinse well with tepid water.

A simple dry mask can be made from a mixture of clays such as Fuller's earth and kaolin and water. Apply a thin layer to the face and allow to dry. Clay masks are very good at drawing oils and impurities out of the skin. Remember when using any type of mask to apply to clean skin and to avoid putting it on the delicate skin around the eyes. Avoid any areas where there are broken veins.

- **Moisturise**. You don't need complicated mixtures to moisturise your skin. Simple oils work just fine. Natural vegetable oils are more compatible with the skin, much less drying than mineral oils and better absorbed than either mineral oil or silicones. Good examples include almond, coconut, jojoba, soya, carrot, wheatgerm, macadamia, olive and avocado. Some animal-derived oils such as squalene and emu also make good alternatives. These oils are more than just vehicles for other ingredients; they often have skin-boosting qualities of their own, for instance they are high in essential fatty acids and Vitamins A, D and E. These fatty acids temporarily strengthen cell membranes, slowing down the formation of fine lines and wrinkles and helping the skin to resist attack from free radicals. Beeswax and soya wax are good alternatives to silicones, while vegetable glycerine and honey are effective, natural humectants.

Lips

Lips are prone to losing moisture quickly, especially in dry atmospheres. This is because lips lack melanin (the body's natural protective hormone against sun damage) and the sebaceous glands which produce natural oils that keep skin supple elsewhere. This makes them prone to moisture loss, chapping and cracking, which in turn can raise the risk of infections like cold sores.

Natural oils and waxes (for instance beeswax or a soya-based wax) are great for everyday wear and can help make an effective barrier to keep lips moist. In addition try these natural lip treatments:

- When you **wash your face** don't forget your lips. Gentle exfoliation with a damp flannel or microfibre cloth can help remove dead skin cells.
- **Vitamin therapy**. Rub the contents of a Vitamin E capsule on your lips and leave overnight for a healing and nourishing treatment.

- **Make your own lip balm**. You'll need 10ml (2tsp) Vitamin E oil (*tocopherol*), 50ml (5tbsp) jojoba oil, 10g (½oz) beeswax and ½ teaspoon honey (optional). Mix oils together. Melt the beeswax slowly in a bain-marie. Add the oils and honey, keeping the mixture over the heat and beat well until the ingredients are thoroughly blended. This moisture can then be poured into a small jar and left to set.
- **For cold sores**. Essential oils have antiviral and antibacterial properties and can help relieve pain and speed healing of cold sores. Try mixing 5 drops each of lavender, geranium and tea-tree essential oil with 1tbsp myrrh tincture. Pour into a bottle and shake to mix. Apply sparingly throughout the day.

Acne treatments

Acne is a common skin disease that affects individuals of all ages. It is largely self-limiting (i.e. it eventually clears up whether you do anything

EYECARE

The skin around your eyes is very delicate and highly reactive to stress, tiredness and polluted atmospheres. A good way to help reduce puffiness is to gently pat the bone around the eye with your middle finger. Alternatively, you can put a couple of stainless steel spoons in the freezer for about 10 minutes and then place them over the eyes for a few minutes to cool and refresh the eye area. Other ways to look after your eyes include:

- **Use witch hazel.** Keep a bottle in the fridge and when your eyes feel puffy, soak cotton pads in the liquid and apply to closed eyes for a few minutes.
- **Make a nourishing eye oil.** Try mixing 30ml (2tbsp) jojoba oil and 30ml (2tbsp) rosehip oil in a small bottle. Using a finger, apply a drop or two with a patting motion to clean damp skin. Leave for 10–20 minutes then blot off any remaining oil. This will both cleanse and moisturise which means you don't need to invest in special eye creams.

about it or not) and most common in teenagers, affecting 80–95 per cent of adolescents at some point and to varying degrees. Teenagers often use antibacterial products believing that they contain some sort of magic that will wash away spots. They won't. Typically such products contain:

- **Benzoyl peroxide**. An antibacterial that can cause contact dermatitis and sensitisation.
- **Salicylic acid**. A chemical exfoliant that can cause skin dryness, irritation, increases skin sensitivity to sunlight (photosensitization) and acts as a penetration enhancer.
- **Harsh detergent/surfactants** such as *sodium laureth sulphate* (*SLES*) which can be contaminated with the carcinogen *1,4-dioxane*, and/or the potential hormone-disrupters *cocamide DEA* and *triethanolamine* (*TEA*).
- **PEG**, or *polyethylene glycol*, compounds are preservatives that can be contaminated with the carcinogen *1,4-dioxane*. *PEGs* can also form carcinogens when mixed with *DEA* and *TEA*. *Pareth* is a surfactant that also belongs to the same family as *polyethylene glycol*.
- **Phenoxyisopropanol** is an antibacterial agent. It is manufactured by combining carcinogenic *phenol* (coal tar) with the solvent *isopropanol*. It is an irritant and allergic reactions are a possible side-effect of use.
- **Carbomer** is a gelling agent that can be irritating to skin and eyes.
- **Parfum** does not clean the face and can be a source of skin and airway irritation.
- **Colour** does not clean the skin and is added only to make the product look nicer.

Spots are most often a result of hormones and poor lifestyle. Plenty of sleep, water in favour of soft drinks, cutting down on sugar and fat, investigating food or other allergies (if the problem is really severe) and a little patience is the best way to tackle them.

Consider these alternative approaches to supporting your skin while your body tackles your spots from the inside:

- **Forget about antibacterial cleansers**. Simple soap and warm water are among the best antibacterials and most effective ways to keep your face clean. They are also less expensive and unlikely to have as many suspect chemicals in them.

- **Try a honey facial**. Use manuka honey for its antibacterial properties and to dissolve dead skin cells. Simply spread over the face and leave for 15 minutes. Rinse with warm water and pat dry.

Although it sounds like a cliché, beauty really is more than skin deep. So many aspects of our lifestyles affect how we look. Likewise, how we feel about ourselves, how confident or stressed, how happy or unhappy we are can be reflected in our faces, in the way we carry ourselves. This in turn has a lot to do with what we project to the outside world. Learning to read labels and to cut out toxic toiletries is an important part of any good beauty routine, but it must be seen as part of a whole lifstyle shift that includes simply learning to love yourself, whoever you are!

Chapter 9
Bath Soaps and Body Washes

Once upon a time, a simple bar of soap was all we needed to get clean. But take a look around the bathroom at all the cleansing products we use now – body washes, bath foams, baby wash and shower gels, facial washes and scrubs. Just how dirty do we think we are?!

Today, most of us do not use soap at all which is a shame because soap is a simple, effective and largely natural cleanser. It is a simple substance made in a one-step process (to make a basic soap all that is required is fat or oil and a strong alkali solution) that creates little waste in its manufacture and little waste in its use. Instead, we use bath bars made from a mixture of different detergents. Unlike soap, detergents, though they may be commonly known as 'soap', can only be produced synthetically in an energy-intensive process and can be harsh on skin, hair and eyes.

Both detergents and surfactants are produced from either plant materials or petrochemicals. Amazingly, there is no difference between the detergents that are in your household cleaning products and those that you use in your bath. It is simply a matter of concentration.

Detergents, which replaced simple soap in our hygiene routines soon after WWII and which form a major part of most bath products, were originally developed for industrial use in hard-water areas where they were thought to clean more efficiently. Since then, research has shown

LIFTING THE LID

The difference between soap and detergent is rather like the difference between cotton and nylon. Soap and cotton are produced from natural products by a relatively small modification. However, detergents and nylon are produced entirely in a chemical factory. Detergents have a greater impact on the environment than soaps, both from the waste stream they generate during their manufacture and due to their poorer biodegradability.

that simple soap and detergent perform equally effectively in most types of waters, although hard water appears to increase the potential of both types of cleaners to irritate the skin.

Manufacturers also boast that, unlike soap, detergents do not produce 'precipitate' – that scummy substance that floats on the water or sticks to the side of the bath or shower. This is not strictly true; all washing products produce some degree of precipitate.

The problem can occur during the rinse. In hard-water areas, both types of cleaners can be difficult to wash off; but old-fashioned soaps even more so. However, genuine castile soap, made with a high percentage of coconut oil, appears to rinse equally well in both types of water.

Having said this, even among detergents there is a great variation in effectiveness and ecological impact. Those based on plant materials are somewhat kinder to the body and environment than those based on petroleum. While for some industrial applications a harsh detergent is an appropriate choice, it is unnecessary for human hygiene.

When you buy detergent-based body-care products it is possible to make safer choices by choosing those made with ingredients that have a milder action on the skin and/or which don't contain potential carcinogens (see Appendix 1).

Bath bars

That good old bar in the bath or shower is the mainstay of most people's personal-care regime. While conventional bath bars are not the worst things you can use on you body, many have the potential to dry and irritate skin.

Most bath bars are made from synthetic and semi-synthetic detergents including *sodium tallowate* – made from animal fats – and *sodium palmate*, *sodium palm kernelate* and *sodium cocoate* which, although of vegetable origin, can be highly processed and retain none of their original vegetable characteristics. They can also contain glycerine (a humectant), water softeners such as *pentasodium disodium EDTA* and *tetrasodium EDTA*, skin conditioners such as stearic acid, rinse aids such as sodium chloride as well as parfum and synthetic colours.

They may all look the same and largely contain the same ingredients, but manufacturers claim significant differences with regard to the degrees of effectiveness and mildness between their products. There is some basis for such claims. For example, glycerine-based soaps are among the mildest on the market, while deodorant and antibacterial soaps are among the harshest and most irritating to skin.

If you want to choose the mildest and most effective bar of soap look for those that contain only vegetable-based ingredients and which don't have any colours in them. If they have organic certification all the better, since these soaps will have minimal preservatives in them and use essential oils instead of heavy synthetic perfumes as a fragrance.

CARING FOR DRY SKIN

You don't need soap to have a wash. If your skin is very dry or irritated, try making your own herbal wash bag. Cut the foot off of an old pair of tights, about 15cm (6 in) from the end. Fill the pouch with a handful of oatmeal, some soothing herbs such as chamomile or lavender and 30ml (2tbsp) of finely ground almonds. Tie a knot in the open end of the pouch. You can now use this in the bath or shower. One wash bag will last one day maximum – keep it in the fridge in a plastic bag if you intend to use it morning and night, but don't try to store it longer than this as it can accumulate bacteria. When wet it will produce a lovely creamy liquid that will clean and nourish your skin without drying it. This is great for adults, babies and children with dry skin.

Bubble baths and body washes

Of all the available bath products, bubble baths, which are highly fragranced, have the greatest potential to cause skin irritation, allergic skin reactions and headaches. However, a bigger problem with using bubble baths is that they can irritate more than just your skin. Regular use is associated with a high rate of urinary tract infections. The harsh detergents in these products can strip away protective oils from sensitive areas of skin as well as stripping away the mucous which lines the genito-urinary tract. Removing this natural protection allows bacteria to take hold. Children are particularly vulnerable and bubble baths are a major cause of urogenital infections in babies.

The mildest and most effective soaps contain only vegetable-based ingredients

Body washes come in liquids, gels and foams but essentially they are the same product as a bubble bath. Soaking in any kind of bath product may be just what you long for after a hectic day, but it will prolong its contact with your skin. Hot water also increases your skin's permeability and helps vaporise some of the chemicals in the product so that they are more easily inhaled. So both bubble baths and shower gels have the potential to get inside your body through your skin and lungs.

Your bubble bath or shower foam is likely to contain detergents like *sodium laureth sulphate* and *cocamidopropyl betaine*, preservatives such as *tetrasodium EDTA, methylchloroisothiazolinone* and *methylisothiazolinone*, and humectants such as *propylene glycol* or *butylene glycol*. If your bubble bath has *cocamide DEA* (or similar compounds ending with *DEA, TEA* or *MEA*) along with formaldehyde-forming substances such as *2-bromo-*

LIFTING THE LID

In America, bubble baths are now obliged to carry a health warning advising users to follow directions carefully and that prolonged use can cause skin irritation and raise the risk of urinary tract infections.

2-nitropropane-1,3-diol (*bronopol* or *BNP*), *DMDM hydantoin, diazolidinyl urea, imidazolidinyl urea* and *quaternium 15* there is the possibility it contains cancer-causing nitrosamines (see Appendix 1 for more details).

A chemical-free alternative

It might come as a shock, but most bath products are unnecessary. Anything that produces a lot of foam has been made to appeal to your emotions and senses, rather than to your desire to be clean, since foam possesses no cleaning ability. However, manufacturers constantly add more detergent and additional foam boosters to produce the foam that they believe consumers can't possibly live without. The increased concentration of detergent creates the need for conditioners and other additives that generate a much more complex cocktail of ingredients in the attempt to limit any skin reaction to the detergents.

The best alternative is to stick to bath bars, avoid bubble baths altogether and limit your use of bath foams and shower gels. If you are looking for the mildest way to clean your skin then:

- **Always opt for vegetable- and glycerine-based detergents** over harsher petrochemical-based varieties.
- **Buy real soap** made from at least 70 per cent vegetable oil. Many health food shops stock them or you can order them from specialist suppliers (see Resources).
- **Choose a liquid castile soap** instead of a body wash. Liquid castile soaps (such as those made by Dr Bronner) foam beautifully and are made from enriching oils such as coconut, hemp and olive. They are usually fragranced with essential oils (but check the label) and even come unscented so you can add your own fragrance.
- **If you must have bubble baths** take them less often and make sure your bathroom is well-ventilated to avoid inhaling too great a concentration of chemicals.

If you are feeling more ambitious, making your own bath products means you can have exactly the right scent to suit your mood on any given day. It also ensures that you are not soaking in or inhaling a bathtub full of potentially harmful chemicals.

- **Use essential oils** to fragrance your bath. To help them disperse in the water mix 4–10 drops of essential oil in 15ml (1tbsp) of milk (semi-skimmed or whole). The fat in the milk will distribute the oils evenly around the bath. Alternatively, mix in a carrier oil such as almond or grapeseed. See the box on page p. 93 for suggestions of the best essential oils to use.

- **A fragrant mineral bath**. No need to buy expensive brands. Add a generous handful of Epsom salts and a few drops of your favourite essential oil (mixed in a carrier as above). Epsom salts can be purchased at chemists in large bags for a minute fraction of the cost of brands that are essentially the same thing. You can add a handful of bicarbonate of soda for some fizz. Epsom salts are a good way of encouraging the skin to release accumulated toxins, so in addition to being pleasant and safe to soak in, they are therapeutic as well.

- **Make your own bathbomb**. Commercially made bathbombs may contain dubious chemicals and colours. Instead, if you want your bath to fizz nicely, mix 45mg (3tbsp) bicarbonate of soda with 22mg (1½tbsp) of citric acid in a bowl together with 8–10 drops of your favourite essential oil. Drizzle a scant teaspoon of water over the dry ingredients and mix well. This is enough for one large bath bomb. You can press it into a mould (an old film cartridge or an ice tray will do) and store in a plastic bag for later. Or you can use it right away by sprinkling the mixture in the bath just as you are getting in.

- **Have a herbal bath**. Brew up a strong infusion of your favourite herbal tea and mix this into your bath water. Good choices include peppermint, chamomile, lavender and limeflower.

- **Make your own body wash**. Liquid castile soap is very versatile and can be combined with other ingredients to make your own personally blended body wash. For a superb cleansing wash, try putting 60ml (4tbsp) castile soap in a bottle and blending with 10ml (2tsp) of Fuller's earth (available from most chemists), 10ml (2tsp) of almond oil and 20 drops of the essential oil(s) of your choice. Remember to shake well before using. If your skin is very dry omit the Fuller's earth. Because this mixture does not contain water, it will last indefinitely.

- **Dry skin brushing**. An effective way to encourage good circulation and to gently exfoliate is to regularly brush your body all over with a natural bristle brush. Dry skin brushing also stimulates the flow of lymph via the lymph vessels. Lymph is a watery substance that helps remove waste from the body whose healthy flow is a sign of a healthy immune system. Always use long strokes in an upward direction towards the heart.

- **Make your own body scrub**. In a bowl or other wide-mouthed container mix 90ml (6tbsp) finely ground salt or sugar (salt works best for oily skin; sugar for normal to dry) with 200ml (7floz) of vegetable oil (olive, almond or grapeseed are good choices). Essential oils are optional. Apply to damp skin and rinse well. It will leave your skin very soft (but beware it can also make the tub or shower quite slippery).

WHICH ESSENTIAL OIL?

When you are ready to try making your own products, use the following guidelines to choose essential oils that match your skin type.

- **Greasy skin:** Lavender, orange, lemon, clary sage, neroli, cypress, ylang ylang, bergamot.
- **Normal skin:** Palma rosa, geranium, lavender, Roman chamomile, jasmine, neroli, ylang ylang, frankincense, sandalwood, patchouli.
- **Sensitive skin:** Geranium, lavender, German chamomile.
- **Dry or damaged skin:** Geranium, lavender, German chamomile, Roman chamomile, clary sage, naiouli, thyme, myrrh or a mixture of eucalyptus and lemon or peppermint.

Chapter 10

Hair Care

How many different types of shampoo have you tried in your lifetime? And how often have they fallen short of what they promised to do?

The main function of a shampoo is to clean the hair. Its function is so simple that advertisers have to work doubly hard to make it sound more complicated and exciting than it actually is. Thus using a particular brand brings with it the promise of harmony, lust for life, nourishment and adoration by members of the opposite sex. Some shampoos are apparently so remarkable that they not only clean your hair but give you an orgasm as well! But underneath all the puffery, a shampoo is just a bottle of highly coloured, highly perfumed detergent.

If you have had more than your share of shampoo disappointments it could be because of unrealistic expectations of what shampoo can achieve. Likewise it could be because there are only a limited number of cleansing agents considered suitable for use in hair cleaning products. If you are unsure of the truth of this statement, compare the labels of expensive designer brands with their cheaper cousins. Often the only genuine difference between them is the price.

The word shampoo is derived from 'chapo', a Hindi word meaning to massage or knead. The first shampoos were simple soap solutions invented by British hairdressers during the heyday of the Empire. Modern shampoos, however, are usually a mixture of several different detergents and surfactants, typically *sodium lauryl sulphate*, *ammonium lauryl sulphate*, *monoethanolamine (MEA) lauryl sulphate*, *diethanolamine (DEA) lauryl sulphate*, and *triethanolamine (TEA) lauryl sulphate*.

Generally, the strongest detergent is used in the greatest measure. Then milder detergents/surfactants, which modify the harshness of the first detergent, are added. These other detergents/surfactants can also add foaming ability and conditioning properties.

For the formulator, the choice of detergent for any particular shampoo is as much a matter of aesthetics as it is cleaning. For instance, *sodium lauryl sulphate* is not very soluble in cold water and so it cannot be used to make shampoos that look 'clear'. For these shampoos other compounds such as *ammonium lauryl sulphate* or *TEA lauryl sulphate* are used. Some shampoos have extra ingredients in them to make them produce more foam, which makes them feel more luxurious but doesn't actually do anything to clean your hair.

Carcinogens in the mix

As detailed in Chapter 3, a number of common ingredients in detergent-based products – such as *2-bromo-2-nitropropane-1,3-diol* (also called *bronopol* or *BNP*), *DMDM hydantoin*, *diazolidinyl urea*, *imidazolindinyl urea* and *quaternium 15* – break down into formaldehyde during storage. When formaldehyde-forming agents mix with amines, e.g. *diethanolamine (DEA)*, *triethanolamine (TEA)* and *monoethanolamine (MEA)*, they form carcinogenic *N-nitrosodiethanolamine (NDELA)*.

A further problem is that products containing the milder *laureth* detergents (as in *sodium laureth sulphate* and *ammonium laureth sulphate*)

LIFTING THE LID

Nitrosamine formation is particularly problematical in shampoos since we use them so frequently and in such great quantities. It is estimated that when you wash your hair with a shampoo contaminated with *NDELA* your body absorbs more carcinogenic nitrites than if you had eaten a pound of bacon!

LIFTING THE LID

Shampoo ingredients can build up on hair over time. To get rid of shampoo build-up, once a week, try rinsing your hair through with ½ cup of bicarbonate of soda or half a cup of white vinegar mixed with 1 cup of warm water. Follow with a thorough rinse with plenty of water.

can be contaminated with the carcinogen *1,4-dioxane*. *Laureth* compounds are part of a larger family of chemicals called ethoxylated alcohols. Many of these, including *polyethylene glycol (PEG), polyethylene, polyoxyethylene, oxynol* and other 'eth' chemicals can be contaminated with *1,4-dioxane*. Products containing *polysorbates 60* and *80* can also be contaminated with this chemical.

The contamination of the raw materials used to create *sodium laureth sulphate* was noted as far back as 1978 and has been confirmed in recent studies. Yet little has been done to address this issue.

As manufacturers fall over themselves to make more 'scientific' and 'improved' shampoos, the list of chemical ingredients grows. The latest published research reveals that the preservatives *methylchloroisothiazolinone* and *methylisothiazolinone* (which together are sometimes called Kathon CG) have the potential to cause nerve damage and skin cancer.

Using nice hot water to shampoo your hair actually increases the rate of absorption of these chemicals into your body, for instance through your skin or by inhaling them in a steamy atmosphere, so if you don't like cold showers, choose your shampoos carefully.

Conditioners

Have you ever noticed how shampoo bottles always recommend that you use a conditioner afterwards? This is because the detergents used in shampoos can be so harsh that you need to use a conditioner to repair some of the damage done by their use. Healthy hair rarely needs conditioning. Hair damaged by detergent use (and other assaults like heated tongs, rollers and styling products) almost always does.

All shampoos, no matter how 'mild', will strip away the protective layer of sebum (natural oils produced by the scalp) that coats your hair. Stripping the sebum away exposes the outside layer of the hair, known as the cuticle. The cuticle is made up of translucent overlapping cells that are arranged like the tiles on a roof. When these cells are disturbed they can rub against each other and become damaged, resulting in the social horror of flyaway hair. Stripping away the sebum also leaves the cortex (the inner part of the hair shaft) vulnerable to damage from other chemicals used on the hair.

Many shampoos contain conditioning agents that smooth down the cuticle and cover it with a synthetic version of sebum. Conditioners, whether they are used separately or incorporated into your regular shampoo, do not repair hair. They cannot penetrate the hair shaft and make it stronger. Instead they coat the hair with chemicals that temporarily 'glue' the damaged hair shaft down, giving the illusion of smoother hair.

A typical hair conditioner will contain surfactants like *triethanolamine* (*TEA*), film formers like *polyvinylpyrrolidone* (*PVP*) and various silicones such as *dimethicone*, humectants like *propylene glycol* and glycerine, *quaternium* compounds, preservatives like *DMDM hydantoin*, *disodium EDTA*, *methylchloroisothiazolinone* and *methylisothiazolinone*. They also contain *parfum*.

The most sensible alternative is not to use a conditioner at all. If you follow the advice below for using or making milder shampoos you should not need a conditioner.

STOP FLYAWAY HAIR

Jojoba oil lubricates, improves shine and lustre, restores damaged hair, strengthens the hair shaft and treats scalp imbalances. If the weather is dry or windy or your hair is a bit flyaway, put two or three drops onto your hands, rub them together and then through the ends of your hair for quick conditioning.

Try this instead

Hair care begins with what you eat, not what you wash with. Hair is 95 per cent protein so if your hair is limp consider whether your protein intake is adequate.

Hair also needs to be thoroughly wet before shampooing. This helps to spread the shampoo evenly throughout the hair. For really clean hair you need to rinse thoroughly, but in the 'wash and go' culture this is a step which most of us rush through. In addition:

- **Read the label**. It really is worthwhile finding a shampoo with the fewest possible ingredients in order to limit your exposure to harmful chemicals. Don't buy products that contain formaldehyde-forming agents and *amines* (ingredients with the letters *TEA*, *MEA* or *DEA* in the name).
- **Use less**. Sounds obvious, but most of us use far too much shampoo to get the job done. A single shampoo using half what you normally use will clean your hair perfectly well. Always tip your head well back when rinsing to avoid any getting onto your eyelids and into your eyes.

You can't make a shampoo based on all natural ingredients. At some point you will have to add detergent – which is always a synthetic ingredient (though some are less harsh and less harmful to the environment than others). But you can adapt the products that you buy to make them less concentrated and so expose yourself to fewer harmful chemicals in each wash. So:

- **Dilute it**. Mix your shampoo with an equal amount of water and put this mixture in an old and well-rinsed shampoo bottle. Adding a little bit of table salt (5ml (1tsp) per 100ml 3½floz) of liquid) will help to thicken the mixture.

  For a variation on the diluting theme, try this: Half fill an old shampoo bottle with your regular shampoo. Top up with an equal amount of water or a strong herbal infusion (such as chamomile) mixed with 5ml (1tsp) of coconut oil (this comes as a solid but can be melted in the hot infusion). Olive or jojoba oils are also good choices. Add 5–10ml (1–2tsp) of table salt to thicken or alternatively

5–10ml (1–2tsp) of sodium bicarbonate to help soften the water and aid rinsing (dissolve this in the water/tea mixture before mixing). This mixture will still foam well and will clean and condition your hair too. Always give it a shake before using, as the ingredients in some shampoo mixtures will separate when the mix is altered.

- **Use a castile soap**. These come in both bar and liquid form. Because of their high oil content, castile soaps will wash and condition your hair. Alternatively, use a pure vegetable oil soap (these can usually be found at specialist suppliers). These types of soaps can also be used on the body, thus saving you money as well as being safer.
- **Use a shampoo bar**. Solid formulations require fewer preservatives and emulsifiers and also use less packaging. Many manufacturers of natural and organic beauty products now offer a shampoo bar as an alternative.

If you wish to continue to use conventional conditioners, once again the best advice is to use less. You can do this in two ways. First, only use a conditioner once or twice a week. Second, you can put less on your hair at each washing. This can be hard to do straight from the bottle so try diluting it instead. To do this, half fill a well-rinsed conditioner bottle with regular conditioner and then top up with water. Shake before use. Alternatively, consider some more basic alternatives:

- **Regular trimming** and keeping the use of hair-destroying stuff like rollers, curling irons, hairdryers and lots of drying styling gels to a minimum will also help keep hair looking good and prevent it from drying out.
- **Condition before you wash**. Contrary to what we have been encouraged to believe, this is the best way to keep hair soft and manageable. Rubbing some good quality oil through your hair half an hour or so before you shampoo, or better still at night before bed, will provide the same conditioning action as the complex and hazardous ingredients in your usual conditioner. Good choices for conditioning oils include olive oil for deep conditioning and coconut, jojoba or almond oil for light to medium conditioning. Add 30ml (2tbsp) of honey to 100ml (3½ floz) oil to help improve the appearance of split ends. Leave on for 30 minutes before shampooing.

DRY HAIR DAY?

If your hair seems a bit dry, try rubbing a few drops of a natural oil into it. Rub two or three drops of a light oil, such as almond or apricot kernel oil, onto damp hands and then run your fingers through the ends of your hair to keep flyaway hair at bay.

Anti-dandruff shampoos

Anti-dandruff shampoos are made with detergents to which anti-flaking agents, such as coal tar, *zinc pyrithizone, salicylic acid* and *selenium sulphide* are added. While they can relieve itching and decrease flaking, no dandruff shampoo can control dandruff completely.

Sulphur and *salicylic acid* work by breaking the flakes into smaller, less noticeable pieces. It is thought that coal tar, *selenium sulphide* and *zinc pyrithizone* can slow the production of flakes. Beyond this, there is little known about how exactly anti-dandruff shampoos work.

Of all the anti-flaking agents, *zinc pyrithizone* and coal tar are considered to be the most effective in controlling dandruff. All anti-flaking agents have some side effects. They can be irritating to both skin and eyes. In particular *salicylic acid*, an ingredient of aspirin, can be severely irritating and is a poison if swallowed. Coal tar is a known carcinogen and can be an irritant when inhaled or when it comes into contact with skin.

A chemical-free alternative

- Dandruff is caused by a fungus. It is most effectively treated from within. Effective **dietary measures** include cutting out sugar and yeasty foods, supplementing with B-complex and probiotics (*acidophilous* and *bifidobacterium*) and making sure you drink plenty of water each day.

- Externally, a more natural alternative is to make an **effective anti-dandruff lotion** with 5ml (1tsp) each of rosemary and thyme essential oils mixed in to 100ml (3½floz) of apple juice and 30ml (2tbsp) cider vinegar. Store in a small spray bottle to make an even application easier. Apply this at bedtime or on days when you can let your hair dry naturally to help keep dandruff at bay.

- **Get a head massage**. In Chinese and Indian medicine, as well as in Western therapies like cranial osteopathy, the head is one of the gateways to the body. Massaging the scalp stimulates several internal parts of the body including the nervous and circulatory systems and the glands. It can promote hair growth as well as reduce dandruff.

Styling products

Like shampoos, many of us tend to collect half-used pots, tubes and bottles of this stuff – a good indication that they never quite do what they are supposed to. Apart from hit-and-miss performance, most styling products contain pretty dubious chemicals which your hair, skin and lungs would be better off without.

Hairspray

Hairspray is essentially plastic dissolved in a solvent and put in a pressurised can or pump spray. It works by gluing strands of hair together so that they form a stronger structure that can then hold a style. Recently it has been reported that hairspray also contains *phthalates* – hormone-disrupting chemicals which are used to keep plastics and vinyl soft and pliable.

Many people find it hard to believe that hairspray is just liquid plastic. If you are one of them, try this test. Spray your usual hair spray onto your bathroom mirror and leave it to dry. If you spray it in a thick enough layer you should be able to peel it off in a single sheet once it dries. But even if you don't, you will be able to scrape off little shavings of plastic – the same stuff that you deposit on your hair and into your eyes and lungs each time you use hair spray.

Hairspray also contains other ingredients such as *Alcohol denat, dimethyl ether, VA/vinyl butyl benzoate/crotonates copolymer, aminomethyl propanol, cyclopentasiloxane, dimethicone copolyol, PPG-3 methyl ether* and parfum.

Perhaps unsurprisingly, there is a medical condition known as hairdresser's lung – a respiratory disease caused by chronic exposure to hairspray. Even though the average consumer is unlikely to get this disease, using hairspray regularly can do other nasty things to your health. Your nose is lined with tiny hairs that filter out dirt from the air you breathe. When hairspray gets into your nose and onto these little hairs, they become sticky and begin to attract dust and pollution until they become saturated with dirt, at which point they stop filtering pollutants effectively.

> *When inhaled, hairspray can stop your nose*
> *filtering pollutants effectively*

Other distressing side-effects of hairspray use include nail abnormalities. When you spray and then style your hair using your fingers the spray is deposited on the nail where it can cause the new nail to grow poorly or predispose it to infection. Breathing difficulties and contact dermatitis after hairspray use are also common.

Hair gel

Like hairspray, hair gel is a type of resin or plastic. Hair gels are generally more concentrated than hairsprays, which is why you can use them to make your hair stick in so many different gravity-defying shapes. Common ingredients include *polyvinylpyrrolidone (PVP)*, *PVP/dimethyl-aminoethylmethacrylate copolymer*, *laureth-23*, *triisopropanolamine*, *carbomer*, *methicone copolymer*, *polyquaternium 4*, *propylene glycol*, preservatives such as parabens, *DMDM hydantoin*, *disodium EDTA*, *diazolidinyl urea*, *phenoxyethanol*, perfume and even synthetic colours.

LIFTING THE LID

Most hair styling products are used to make up for poor-quality cuts and years of abusive practices such as using harsh shampoos, hair dryers, heated rollers and styling wands. The best solution could be to spend the money you normally spend on styling products on a really good haircut. With a really good haircut you should not need to apply lots of glue to your hair to keep it in place. Do this and you may find that you and your hair live happily ever after.

Styling foam

Most styling foams or mousse are made from a combination of water, film-forming resins, surfactants and a propellant system. Fixatives like *polyquaternium-4*, solvents like *propylene glycol*, plasticisers like *C9-C11 Pareth-8*, and preservatives such as *DMDM Hydantoin* or *Disodium EDTA* can most often be found in styling foams. Apart from providing a bit of hold to our style, mousse products traditionally have a strong element of conditioning associated with them, along with other properties such as easy wet combing, good holding power, better volume, shine and a smooth, silky feel on hair. But the 'conditioning' provided by your mousse is an artifice – the resins and plastics in them may make your hair feel smoother in the short term, but they do nothing to actually improve the condition of your hair. In fact, the more you use them the more these ingredients can build up on your hair, decreasing its volume and making it dull and unattractive. Adding 'nutrients' such as panthenol are unlikely to remedy this.

Hair mousse also has certain things in it that the styling lotions of old didn't. Atmosphere-damaging propellants such as *isobutane*, *butane* and *propane* are common. These propellants may not destroy the earth's ozone shield, but they do contribute to the formation of ground-level ozone, or smog, which can cause serious respiratory problems.

Because they are based on water they also contain a range of skin, irritating preservatives. To keep it all mixed together, industrial strength solvents are added, such as *propylene glycol* – which is used in anti-freeze. Styling foams are also often very heavily perfumed even though the fragrance portion adds nothing to the performance of the products.

Try this instead

Apart from not using it, there are really very few alternatives to things like hairspray, gel and mousse. So if you don't want to stop using these products entirely, try reserving them for when you really need them, like on special occasions. When purchasing hairsprays, gels and other styling agents:

- **Read the label**. Try to buy products with the fewest and least-toxic ingredients.

- **Choose pump sprays** over aerosols. You are still at risk of inhaling the noxious chemicals in the mixture, but you will be avoiding inhaling toxic propellants as well – a small step in the right direction.

Hair dyes

In a culture obsessed with youth and beauty, grey hairs are the enemy and today's hair dyes are marketed as being as good for your self-esteem as they are for your hair. But underneath the advertising hype is a disturbing amount of data linking regular hair dye use with a range of different cancers.

To achieve luscious shades of chestnut brown, coppery red, mahogany or black, permanent hair dyes must first chemically damage your hair. Under a microscope, the cuticle of human hair looks like overlapping fish scales. The pigment molecules that give hair its colour are stored in the cortex of the hair, beneath this scaly layer. Before the

HAIR REMOVAL

Depilatories, which come in gels, creams, lotions, aerosols and roll-ons are chemical razor-blades. Usually they contain a highly alkaline chemical such as *calcium thioglycolate* which dissolves the protein structure of the hair, causing it to separate from the skin surface. The problem is that skin and hair are similar in their composition. What damages one can also damage the other. For this reason, if you are going to use depilatory creams it is particularly important to follow the directions, not leave them on for longer than recommended and not re-apply too regularly.

Waxing products use a mixture of natural and synthetic waxes, sugars and acids such as citric acid. While their ingredients are usually less alarming than hair removal creams, the process of ripping hair out of the skin by its roots is a violent one that can leave delicate skin irritated. In some instances it is worth pausing to ask yourself why you feel the need to subject yourself to such intense depilation. Are advertising and beauty magazines pressurising you?

colour can penetrate the hair shaft, the cuticle must be 'opened' so that chemicals can get into the natural pigment molecules.

Permanent hair dyes consist of a two components – colour and developer. The colour component usually contains a range of synthetic dyes and intermediates such as ammonia, *diaminobenzenes*, *phenylenediamines*, *resorcinol* and *phenols*.

Mixed with the developer – usually hydrogen peroxide – the colour component begins to oxidise to produce a particular colour. The ammonia in the mix causes the hair shaft to swell, forcing the cuticles apart and allowing the mix to deposit the new colour underneath. The process of oxidation takes time, which is why the formula usually looks one colour when you first apply it and another when your rinse it off.

Toxic ingredients like *diaminotoulene* and *diaminoanisole* were removed from hair dye products some 20 years ago but it is likely that past use of dyes containing these chemicals is a cause of some cases of breast cancer today. Even so, a quick label scan of most hair dyes today reveals the names of chemicals, most commonly *phenylenediamines*, which are just as harmful. The type of *phenylenediamine* used depends on the end colour:

- *para-phenylenediamine* (black)
- *para-toluenediamine* (brown)
- *ortho-phenylenediamine* (brown)
- *para-aminophenol* (reddish brown)
- *ortho-aminophenol* (light brown)

Other hair dye ingredients (look out for *4-chloro-m-phenylenediamine*, *2,4-toluenediamine*, *2-nitro-p-phenylenediamine* and *4-amino-2-nitrophenol*) have also proven carcinogenic in at least one animal species. Coal-tar dyes have also been found to cause cancer in laboratory animals, yet no warning is required for these either.

These ingredients and their variations (usually *HCl*, *hydrochloride* or sulfates like *para-phenylenediamine sulfate*) are powerful irritants and have been implicated in severe allergic reactions. *Phenylenediamines* are also mutagenic (causing DNA mutations and foetal abnormalities in animal studies). Other irritant ingredients include hydrogen peroxide, *resorcinol* and *1-naphthol*. Hair dye sold in the European Union containing any of these ingredients needs to carry the following warning:

Can cause an allergic reaction. Do not use to colour eyelashes or eyebrows.

In the US, products containing *4-methoxy-m-phenylenediamine* (*4-MMPD, 2,4-diaminoanisole*) must also carry a warning:

Contains an ingredient that can penetrate your skin and has been determined to cause cancer in laboratory animals.

No such warning is required for this ingredient in the EU.

Other hair-dye ingredients such as chlorides are highly irritating to the mucus membranes. Chloride fumes can irritate the lungs and eyes and cause burns or rashes on the skin. Hair colours also contain several penetration enhancers known to aid the absorption of other toxic chemicals into the bloodstream. These can include *propylene glycol*, *polyethylene glycol*, fatty acids such as *oleic*, *palmitic* and *lauric acid* and *isopropyl alcohol* to name but a few.

Mounting evidence

Both human and animal studies show that the body rapidly absorbs the carcinogens and other chemicals in permanent and semi-permanent dyes through the skin during the up to 30 minutes period that dyes can remain on the scalp. So if you use permanent, semi-permanent, shampoo-in or temporary hair colours, you are increasing your toxic load as well as your risk of developing cancer.

> *The chloride fumes in hair dyes can cause*
> *burns or rashes to the skin*

Problems with hair dyes were first noted in the late 1970s when several studies found links between the use of hair dyes and breast cancer. In 1976, one study reported that 87 of 100 breast cancer patients had been long-term hair-dye users.

In 1979, another study found a significant relationship between the frequency and duration of hair-dye use and breast cancer. Women who started dyeing their hair at age 20 had twice the risk of 40-year-olds.

Those at greatest risk were the 50- to 79-year-olds who had been dyeing their hair for years, suggesting that the cancer takes years to develop or that prolonged exposure may increase the risk.

A year later, another study found that women who dye their hair to change its colour, rather than masking greyness, were at a threefold risk of developing breast cancer.

Research continued and in the early 1990s Japanese and Finnish studies again linked hair-dye use with breast cancer. More recently, a jointly funded American Cancer Society and FDA study found a four-fold increase in relatively uncommon cancers, including non-Hodgkin's lymphoma (NHL) and multiple myeloma, among hair-dye users.

A more recent Harvard study suggested that compared to women who had never dyed their hair, women who dyed their hair one to four times a year had a 70 per cent increased risk for ovarian cancer. Women who used hair dye five times or more per year had twice the risk of developing ovarian cancer compared to women who never used hair dye.

As if this wasn't enough, a study in 2001 found a link between long-term hair-dye use and an increased incidence of bladder cancer.

But it is the link with otherwise uncommon cancers that causes the greatest concern, and may well be the best evidence of hair-dye toxicity.

Evidence suggests, for example, that if you use hair dye you may be increasing your risk of NHL and multiple myeloma anywhere from

MEN AT RISK TOO

While women were once the main consumers of hair dye, use among men has increased dramatically in the last few decades, and with it the incidence of once rare cancers. According to the NCI hair dye use is responsible for a 90 per cent increased risk of multiple myeloma (a type of cancer of plasma cells) among men.

This result echoed that of an earlier NCI study which showed that men who had used hair dyes had a two-fold risk for non-Hodgkin's lymphoma and almost double the risk of leukaemia.

two to four times over a non-user. Some researchers even believe that hair dyes may account for as many as 20 per cent of all cases of NHL in women.

Other data from the US National Cancer Institute (NCI) shows that women who used permanent hair dyes had a 50 per cent higher risk for developing NHL and an 80 per cent higher risk of multiple myeloma than non-users.

In this study, other cancer risk factors, such as family history of cancer, cigarette smoking, and herbicide or pesticide exposure did not change the risks calculated for hair-dye use and the risk increased with the number of years of use and for women using black, brown and red colouring products.

As a general rule, the darker the shade of the dye, the higher the risk of breast cancer; thus women who use black, dark brown or red dyes are at the greatest risk.

In fairness, there are problems with studies into hair dye and cancer risk. Some involve small numbers of women working in the cosmetics industry. Historically, this group of women is exposed to the known carcinogens in hair dyes (*diaminotoulene*; *diaminoanisole*; *phenylenediamines*; coal tar dyes, the dioxane found in detergents and solvents; *nitrosamines* and formaldehyde-releasing preservatives) in much greater concentration than the rest of us. However, taken together they point towards an increased overall risk.

Some studies dispute the cancer risk of hair dyes. Nevertheless, it is still believed that long-term hair-dye use may account for as many as 20 per cent of all cases of NHL (the cancer which killed long-term black-hair-dye user Jacqueline Kennedy) in women.

'Minimal' risk?

Hair dye manufacturers continue to defend the safety of their products, suggesting that any risk is 'minimal'. It is true that some studies dispute the cancer risk. One which involved 1,500 men and women hair dye users in San Francisco found no increased incidence of NHL. The weight of the evidence, however, suggests a need for caution.

One difficulty is that there are large variations in the chemical content of hair dyes. This means that when an association is found it is difficult to know which ingredient or mix of ingredients is the culprit.

In addition, cancer is a slow-developing disease in humans. By the time it surfaces, it is difficult to prove beyond a shadow of a doubt that one particular exposure was the cause. Good news for manufacturers who can continue to produce potentially toxic products with impunity and without risk of litigation, but bad news for those of us trying to live a natural, less toxic life.

Try this instead

If you intend to keep dyeing your hair, consider the safer options:

- **Read the label**. If you dye your hair, use the safer alternatives that are currently on the market. These should not contain *phenylenediamines* (though many so-called natural hair colours do). Never buy products that are in any way unclear about their ingredients.
- **Read the label again**. This time look for dyes. Avoid products that use colours like Acid Orange 87, Solvent Brown 44, Acid Blue 168 and Acid Violet 73. These are also carcinogenic.
- **Don't dye your hair too often**. Leave the maximum amount of time in between applications.
- Use an applicator to keep the dye on the roots and away as much as possible from the scalp. Leave hair dyes on the head for the **minimum required time**.
- Hair colorants made entirely from **plant-based ingredients** are the safest choice, however these are few and far between. Pure herbal hair dyes will need to be left in the hair significantly longer than synthetic dyes, but have the advantage of conditioning the hair while they colour.
- **A good haircut** can go a long way to making your hair look great without dyes.
- **Go natural**. In a world of look-alike bleach blondes and unnaturally red redheads you'll probably be the standout.

Chapter 11

Deodorants and Antiperspirants

Deodorants have been around for a long time in one form or another. They are strong perfumes that mask the odour produced by bacteria in your armpits. Later, antiperspirants, which prevent sweat from leaking out of the armpits, were developed. Today there is a huge range of antiperspirants, deodorants and antiperspirant/deodorant combinations on the market, in a variety of formulations including creams, roll-ons, solids and sprays. A quick look at the label will tell you that there isn't a wide difference between the ingredients used in any of them.

Antiperspirants and deodorants typically contain a range of solvents, preservatives, synthetic perfumes and antibacterial agents. These days they even contain moisturisers that claim to keep the skin under your arms looking soft and young. While nobody wants to go around smelling like a compost heap (and nobody enjoys being around someone who does), it's worth asking what price we are paying for trying to stay shower fresh all day long.

Finding an answer to this question became more urgent in 2002 when UK researchers highlighted potential risks associated with preservatives known as *para-hydroxybenzoic acids* (parabens) in deodorants. The researchers found traces of parabens in every single tumour sample taken from a small group of women with breast cancer.

Parabens are used in a wide variety of cosmetics. The scientists suggested that the chemicals had seeped into tissue after being applied to the skin, probably via deodorants. The findings are worrying because parabens are oestrogen mimics and this makes them potential triggers for the growth of human breast tumours.

Before the bad news about parabens came out, it was the aluminium content of antiperspirants that was a major cause of concern. Most antiperspirants contain some form of aluminium, most commonly *aluminium chlorohydrate, aluminium zirconium tetrachlorohydrex GLY, aluminium chloride, aluminium sulphate* and *aluminium phenosulphate.*

The recently acknowledged link between Alzheimer's disease and aluminium has raised a furious debate about whether or not it is safe to put aluminium compounds into deodorants. This is not a question that has benefited from much scientific evaluation. Only one study reports a link between Alzheimer's and a lifetime's deodorant use. No other studies have been conducted that refute or confirm these findings, though it is known than aluminium can be absorbed through the skin.

Other evidence which looked at the incidence of breast cancer among 400 US women suggests it may be the combination of underarm shaving and deodorant use which allows chemicals to seep into breast tissue. In this study women who shaved three times a week and applied deodorant at least twice a week were almost 15 years younger when diagnosed than women who did neither. The researchers suggested that aluminium compounds could act as a breast cancer trigger.

LIFTING THE LID

We still don't know exactly how aluminium compounds work to reduce underarm wetness. They may prevent sweat by clogging sweat ducts. Clogging the sweat ducts creates pressure from the sweat build-up inside of them and it is thought that this causes the sweat glands to stop secreting. Alternatively they may perforate the sweat glands so that moisture seeps out into the surrounding tissues rather than coming out through the surface of the skin. Or they may block the transmission of the nerve impulses that activate sweat glands.

NATURAL DEODORANTS

Rock crystals are the newest 'alternative' to aluminium-containing antiperspirants Some of these are made from magnesium sulphate while others are made from alum. These products often claim to be 'aluminium free' or 'free of *aluminium chlorohydrate*', yet alum by its other name is aluminium sulphate. Manufacturers suggest that aluminium sulphate has a much higher molecular weight than *aluminium chlorohydrate* – which is true – and so cannot be absorbed through the skin. However, this may be simplistic. While *aluminium chlorohydrate* has a lower molecular weight, it is also less soluble in water (sweat).

Sulphates on the other hand are highly soluble in water and alum may break down into its component parts more readily in a sweaty armpit. Does this mean that the aluminium will be absorbed into the skin? Without the emollient ingredients found in most conventional formulations it is unlikely, but it would be reassuring if there were more conclusive research evidence to prove that this was true.

Certainly, aluminium-based deodorants are a major cause of skin irritation and for this reason alone should be approached with caution. Prolonged use of *aluminium zirconium* products have been shown to cause granulomas (small nodules of chronically inflamed tissue) under the arms.

Try this instead

Body odour is largely caused by bacteria in your armpits but it can also be caused by what's inside your body, for instance, what you eat and how 'polluted' your body is by toxins and allergens. A healthy, 'unpolluted' body tends to produce less pungent body odour than an unhealthy one.

If you can, try to avoid aluminium-based antiperspirants. The toxicity of aluminium is well established and there is too little evidence of the safety of aluminium-containing products that are applied to the skin. The presence of ingredients such as magnesium oxide and zinc oxide will buffer the irritant properties of aluminium- and zirconium-based compounds, but they too can cause skin irritation.

When selecting conventional antiperspirants and deodorants, consider the following:

- **Avoid aerosols**, which surround you and those in your immediate area with a cloud of easily inhaled and toxic chemicals. Aerosols can contain planet-poisoning HCFCs as well as the neurotoxic and reproductive toxins *propane*, *butane* and *isopropane*, meaning that you may be harming not only yourself, but also the environment, when you use a spray deodorant.
- **Switch to a solid or stick variety**. Because it is less emollient it is less likely to aid the absorption of ingredients into the skin. Sticks also tend to produce less irritation.
- **Never apply antiperspirants or deodorants to broken or newly shaved skin.** The chemicals in them will be much more easily absorbed into your system if your skin is damaged in any way.
- **Avoid coloured products**. The colour will not help you stay drier and the coal tar and petrochemical-derived colours used in these products are easily absorbed into the skin and can be carcinogenic.
- **Avoid products containing *quaternium 18*** which can cause rashes that spread beyond the area of application.

Your healthfood shop may sell deodorants based on plant extracts and essential oils (but remember to read the label to find out what is really in them). Some also sell crystal deodorants made from mineral salts. These can be very effective but always check what they are made of – some are aluminium-based (see box p. 112). Don't buy crystal deodorants whose labels are in any way unclear about the mineral used.

If you are feeling more ambitious you can make your own antiperspirants and deodorants from a few simple ingredients.

Body sprays

Body sprays serve no useful function. They are not deodorants, they are not quite strong enough to be perfumes and they can't stop you from sweating. Nevertheless, the market for body sprays, for men and women, has grown exponentially in recent years.

KEEPING DRY NATURALLY

Dust under your arms with **plain cornstarch**. If you don't sweat heavily this may be all you need.

An equally simple astringent is **witch hazel**, which helps to temporarily contract the tissues around the sweat glands and may be all some people need. Do not apply to broken skin as it may sting.

A mixture of unflavoured **Vitamin C powder** or citric acid and water works well for some people. Mix 1ml (¼tsp) powdered Vitamin C or citric acid with 500ml (1pint) water. Dab this sparingly under your arms after a bath. Or put it in a spray bottle and spritz a little on. If you can't wait for it to dry, dust with cornstarch afterwards.

Try a **'natural deodorant'**. These are widely available in healthfood shops and these days most larger supermarkets have a natural alternative. Natural deodorants are made from or incorporate natural minerals (see box p. 112), but contain no antiperspirants. This means they don't prevent perspiration, which is good, because sweating helps remove unwanted toxins from the body and is necessary for healthy body function. Instead, natural deodorants mask odour with essential oils and the minerals work to inhibit the growth of bacteria that can cause body odour.

For a more ambitious spray, the owners of Neal's Yard, one of the UK's most respected natural toiletry manufacturers, recommend the following:
- 90ml (6tbsp) witch hazel
- 10ml (2tsp) vegetable glycerine
- 2 drops each of clove, coriander and lavender essential oil
- 5 drops each of grapefruit, lime and palmarosa essential oil
- 10 drops of lemon essential oil

Mix the witch hazel and vegetable glycerine together then add the essential oils. Shake well. Store in a dark glass or plastic bottle with a spray top. The mixture will last for up to 6 months.

Advertising for such products suggests that using them will make you more attractive to the opposite sex, or give you the courage to do wild and outrageous things. In reality they are likely to give you a headache (which may stop you from doing wild and outrageous things), cause you to become forgetful, tired and listless and may even make the people around you feel sick.

Body sprays are mostly solvents, propellants and fragrances. The perfumes can cause allergic reactions, headaches, dizziness, fatigue and a range of mental symptoms; the solvents and propellants are neurotoxic and have been implicated in reproductive problems such as miscarriage and birth defects.

A chemical-free alternative

The best alternative is to avoid these unnecessary and expensive items. If you must add yet another fragrance to your body, try to keep it as natural as possible.

SWEATY FEET?

Your feet, like your armpits, contain lots of sweat glands. Hot days, shoes and socks made from synthetic materials can all conspire to make them sweat profusely. Conventional foot deodorants contain all the same ingredients as regular deodorants so you may want to try tackling the problem in a different way. To make a simple foot powder use cornstarch. If you want a powder that perfumes and deodorises, mix 5 drops each of lemon and coriander essential oil in with the cornstarch. Store the perfumed mixture in an old talcum powder dispenser or similar type of container.

For an effective foot deodorant all you need is 30ml (2tbsp) witch hazel and 5 drops each of lavender and grapefruit essential oils. Blend the ingredients together, store in a spray bottle (preferably made of dark coloured glass or plastic). Spray regularly on to clean feet, shaking before applying. This mixture will keep for up to 2 months.

- Use food grade **flower waters**. Rose and orange flower waters can be purchased in your supermarket. While not chemical-free, these have fewer nasties in them than conventional body sprays. Either splash them on to your body directly or transfer to a spray bottle for use.

- You can make a pleasant body spray from **water and essential oils**. Try mixing 5 drops each of lavender, sage, lemon, rosemary and grapefruit essential oils and 3 drops of peppermint into 10ml (2tsp) vodka. Shake to mix. Then add 100ml (3½floz) white vinegar. Leave this mixture to sit for an hour or so to fix the scent. Next add the scented mixture to 500ml (1pint) of spring or filtered water and shake again.

   You can also substitute natural vanilla essence for the essential oils. By learning more about essential oils you can make an infinite number of light splashes and sprays to suit your every mood.

Using talc

Talcum powder is a traditional mainstay of freshness. We use it liberally on babies' bottoms and to absorb perspiration on hot summer days and nights. A few of us are old enough to remember our mothers having special dishes of talc in the bathroom which had big inviting powder puffs to help you dust your body, and most of the bathroom floor, with the stuff.

But time marches on and the romantic illusion of talc has taken a huge knock. Talc (*magnesium silicate*) is made up of finely ground particles of stone. As it originates in the ground, and is a mined product, it can be contaminated with other substances such as asbestos. Recent reports about the talc used in crayon manufacture being contaminated with this poisonous substance have cause alarm to every parent whose child has ever sucked a crayon.

The harmful effects of talc on human tissue were first recorded in the 1930s. More recently a report from the US National Toxicology Program concluded that talc is carcinogenic.

An ominous series of studies has linked talc to ovarian cancer; in them talc was observed in a number of ovarian and uterine tumours as well as in ovarian tissue. It has since been confirmed that talc, either placed directly on the perineum or on the surface of underwear or sanitary towels, can reach the ovaries via ascent through the fallopian tubes. It is now estimated that women who frequently use talc have three times the risk of developing ovarian cancer compared to non-users.

The talc used in the manufacture of condoms carries a similar risk. In the 1960s the medical journal *The Lancet* reported the first case of a woman who had a significant amount of talc in her peritoneal (abdominal) cavity. Laboratory tests confirmed that the talc in her body matched that found on the surface of her husband's condoms. The authors concluded that the talc travelled up through the fallopian tubes and became implanted in her abdomen. Talc sprinkled on diaphragms may also be implicated in such problems.

Talc use is also associated with respiratory problems. Because it is comprised of finely ground stone it can lodge in the lungs and never leave. Babies whose mothers smother them in talc have more breathing difficulties and/or urogenital problems. Women are also at risk since even if they don't use talcum powder on their bodies, they are likely to be using cosmetics (powder, eyeshadow, blusher) that are talc-based.

Feminine deodorants

Feminine deodorants and douches are totally unnecessary. The majority are bought and used simply out of a media-fuelled paranoia which makes women worry that the people around them can detect any faint odours coming from their genitals.

Ironically, the use of feminine deodorants – which are no different from most body sprays – can cause vaginal infections that may be the cause of unpleasant odours. More worryingly, in one study involving nearly 700 women over three years researchers found that women who used vaginal douches more than once a week experienced a four-fold risk of cervical cancer. It did not matter which preparation was used since all douches alter the chemical balance of the vagina, making the cervix more susceptible to bacterial infection and tissue changes.

Feminine deodorants are almost always aerosols, which means that you inhale harmful chemicals when you use them, and they are always highly perfumed. Douches contain harsh detergents, perfumes and colours, none of which should be coming into contact with this delicate area of your body.

TRY THIS INSTEAD

Don't use products containing talc. Giving up body powders is relatively easy. Giving up your eye shadow may be less so (try applying it with a damp sponge to minimise fallout). But whatever you can do to cut your exposure to talc will benefit your health.

- **Make your own.** You can quickly and easily make a very efficient and inexpensive body powder based on cornstarch. Combine one part bicarbonate of soda to eight parts cornstarch. Mix these up in a coffee grinder or blender and add 10–15 drops of your favourite essential oil (optional). Store in an airtight container (either a jar or an old talc container, or you can recycle one of those Parmesan cheese shakers).
- **Babies' bottoms do not need talc** or any other powder to stay fresh. Instead let your baby go without nappies as often as possible, or investigate cotton nappies which allow the skin to breath and have been shown to cause less nappy rash than disposables.
- **Buy talc alternatives**. If you don't want to make your own, a number of manufacturers now make talc-free alternatives that make use of cornstarch and herbs and are fragranced with natural essential oils.
- **Use talc-free condoms,** but be aware. Many talc-free condoms contain other particles such as vegetable starches, silica (another carcinogen), mica and diatomaceous earth and lycopodium (club moss) spores. Lycopodium can be contaminated with talc, sulphur and/or gypsum and is linked with inflammation of soft tissues. It is not known how many chronic 'women's problems' may be the result of over use of talc, or indeed allergy to the latex used in condoms or other contraceptives such as the diaphragm and all the paraphernalia which goes with them (spermicidal jellies, foams, creams and lubricants).

Try this instead

Have a little confidence in yourself and toss these toxic products in the bin where they belong. In addition:

- **Bathe daily**. When you wash your genitals do not apply soap directly. It is too harsh and may dry out delicate skin. Use the foam or bubbles from your soap to gently clean yourself.
- **Wear cotton underwear**, which allows air to circulate and discourages the bacteria that can cause unpleasant odours.
- If you are experiencing vaginal itching or feel you have a problem with strong and unpleasant vaginal odours, **go to your doctor** to sort out the underlying cause of the problem. You may have a low-grade vaginal infection that can easily be cleared up. It is unlikely that it will be something which you can simply wash away with a douche.
- If you must douche, **use a simple mixture** of 10ml (2tsp) distilled white vinegar in one pint of water, which will have less of an impact on the vaginal microflora. Use very infrequently.

Chapter 12
Dental Care

Brushing your teeth several times daily can help keep them clean, clear the mouth of plaque-forming bacteria and freshen the breath. In pursuit of a dazzling smile and a fresh mouth there are now a staggering variety of toothpaste products available including family toothpastes, whitening toothpastes, children's toothpastes, tartar-control toothpastes, toothpastes plus mouthwash, gels, creams and stripes, mild mint, freshmint, baking soda and herbal toothpastes, each one claiming to do something specific and/or unique.

You may think that there's a wide variety of toothpastes on the market, most are basically the same – there is no advantage of using gel toothpaste, for example, over a cream one, and those with stripes don't clean more effectively than those without. And while many toothpastes appear to make grand claims about what they can do for your teeth, look closely at the wording on the label next time you buy. It won't actually say it will prevent plaque or tartar build-up. Instead it says it 'fights it' or 'can help prevent' it. This is a convenient way of sounding like it is making a medicinal claim (and thus gaining the trust of the consumer) when in reality it isn't.

Toothpaste may make your mouth feel fresh, yet it is not actually necessary to clean teeth. Dry brushing can do the job just as effectively.

Specialist toothpastes are also limited in what they can achieve. Tartar-control toothpastes, for example, cannot remove existing tartar. Likewise, those pastes that claim to prevent gum disease cannot treat existing gum disease. In both cases a trip to the dentist is necessary. Smoker's toothpaste, which claims to remove stains, can be highly abrasive. Excessive abrasion on the teeth can damage enamel and cause the gums to recede.

The problems of dental decay and gum disease are very real and impact on more than just the mouth. Periodontal disease has very strong links to other conditions such as heart disease. Indeed, your risk of developing heart disease is much higher if you have poor oral health than if you smoke or have high cholesterol. One theory for why this is suggests that oral bacteria can affect the heart when they enter the bloodstream, attaching to fatty plaques in the coronary arteries (the vessels that deliver blood to the heart) and contributing to clot formation.

Another possibility is that the inflammation caused by periodontal disease increases plaque build-up, which may contribute to swelling of the arteries. Researchers have found that people who have periodontal disease are almost twice as likely to suffer from coronary artery disease as those who don't. Poor oral health also raises your risk of stroke, peripheral vascular disease, osteoporosis, respiratory diseases, diabetes and pre-term pregnancy.

WHAT TYPE OF BRUSH?

Many a weird-shaped toothbrush has been developed over the years, largely to try make up for the lazy way in which most people brush. However, there is very little evidence that they are substantially better than a standard straight-handled brush. What is important for your dental health is the quality of the bristles. Make sure you invest in a brush with lots of filaments packed tightly together. A soft to medium brush is fine for most people (very few really need a firm brush). However, the angle of the head is mostly immaterial. Replace your toothbrush regularly, at the first signs of wear. Some manufacturers now make toothbrushes with replaceable heads. Buying these massively reduces plastic waste.

Nevertheless, brushing, like so many daily tasks, can sometimes be a bit routine, and hence boring. So major manufacturers have begun to advertise toothpaste in a way that suggests it is a beauty or luxury product rather than an aid to personal hygiene. One major brand even promises to provide noticeable improvement for all five signs of healthy teeth – fewer cavities, less tartar, healthy gums, naturally white teeth and fresh breath – in much the same way that anti-wrinkle creams fight the 'seven signs of ageing'.

Hard to swallow

By turning basic daily necessities into more attractive premium purchases, manufacturers can encourage consumers to buy more and pay a higher price. This also has a knock-on effect of drawing attention away from the actual ingredients.

In a market crowded with alternatives, each brand has to make bigger claims about what it can do. And to back up these claims more and more chemicals are added.

Several of the 'active' ingredients in toothpaste are worrying. The industrial-strength detergent *sodium lauryl sulphate* (*SLS*), is a suspected gastrointestinal or liver toxicant. There is also concern that by irritating and stripping away the protective mucous membrane of the mouth, *SLS* could increase the incidence of mouth ulcers and may be implicated in an increased risk of oral cancer.

Triclosan is one of the most common anti-bacterial agents used in toothpaste. It is often found in antibacterial and antiplaque formulas and there is evidence that it can help reduce plaque build-up. But although tartar control formulas may prevent 40–50 per cent of new tartar build-up, they can do nothing for plaque that has already built up.

Like *SLS*, *Triclosan* is an irritant and there is evidence that the two substances can combine synergistically to become even more powerfully irritant. *Triclosan* overuse is also associated with a rise in superbugs, resistant to many kinds of antiseptics and antibiotics.

Certain abrasives found in toothpastes, such as silica, are also potentially harmful. Studies have recently begun to show that fine granules of this mineral can build up under the surface of the gums causing granulomas – small nodules of inflamed tissue. Other fine-grained abrasives can have a similar effect, leading to symptoms that can mimic gingivitis and also leave the gums more vulnerable to infection.

Many toothpastes also contain glue-like substances, such as *PVM/MA copolymer*, that keep the active ingredients in contact with the teeth after rinsing. There is little data on how toxic these plastic glues are if swallowed or absorbed.

Fluoride toothpastes

By far the most controversial ingredient in toothpaste, however, is fluoride. Many of us still buy fluoride-containing toothpastes believing that fluoride protects teeth. There is, however, little convincing scientific evidence of this. Instead, fluoride is a systemic poison. There is enough in the average tube of family toothpaste to kill a small child if ingested. For this reason both the American FDA and the Swedish National Food Administration now require that toothpaste containing fluoride be labelled with a special 'poison' warning.

Studies have shown a clear relationship between oral cancers and fluoride intake in both animals and humans. For instance, benign squamous papilloma, which appears as a white patch on the inside of the mouth and is the precursor of squamous cell carcinoma (a common form of skin cancer), can also be triggered by fluoride exposure.

Fluoride can cause sensitivity and allergic type reactions and is now suspected in a host of illnesses including gastroesophageal reflux disease (GERD), bone problems, diabetes, thyroid malfunction and mental impairment.

LIFTING THE LID

It is now widely accepted that family toothpastes which generally have the highest amounts of fluoride in them (around 1,500ppm, or parts per million) are unsuitable for children under the age of 8. If you are going to buy a fluoride toothpaste for your child, use a children's formula and supervise brushing to make sure it doesn't get swallowed.

Fluoride exposure from toothpaste, supplements and water before the age of six is also an important risk factor for dental fluorisis, which mottles and discolours the teeth. In addition, young children also have a tendency to swallow toothpaste and with it the potentially poisonous fluoride.

More recently, fluoride has been found to activate and interfere with substances known as G-proteins, chemical messengers that play a vital role in the functioning of hormones and neurotransmitters. By activating G-proteins, fluoride may actively promote gingivitis, thus contributing to the whole range of diseases associated with this problem.

Whitening toothpastes

These toothpastes work in two ways, either by bleaching the teeth with chemicals such as hydrogen peroxide (which can be a slow process) or by using gritty particles to rub away stains. Such toothpastes are popular among smokers and those with low self-esteem. The abrasive action is harmful to your teeth. The jury is still out on chemical bleaching. However, problems have already been observed.

At best, whitening toothpastes may produce a mild cleaning or bleaching action that only lasts as long as you keep using the product. At worst they can make your teeth painfully sensitive to heat and cold, may irritate your gums and permanently destroy tooth enamel. Concern has also been expressed that new chemical whiteners are still something of an unknown quantity. Peroxide, for instance, is highly reactive and may interact with other chemicals present in the paste to form new, harmful chemicals.

LIFTING THE LID

Sensitive tooth formulas contain nerve-deadening chemicals such as *strontium chloride* or *potassium nitrate*. Don't expect these toothpastes to work immediately, like they do on TV – most people won't notice any improvement for 4–6 weeks. If your teeth are very sensitive it could be because you are grinding them at night or habitually gritting them. You may, in addition, benefit from a trip to the dentist to rule out an underlying problem, such as a cracked tooth or gum disease.

Mouthwash and breath fresheners

The traditional purpose of a mouthwash is an antiseptic gargle to help remove germs that can lead to bad breath. Today, mouthwashes come in many more complex forms that purport to fight plaque, strengthen teeth, fight tooth decay and freshen breath in addition to killing germs. The more claims the product makes, the more chemicals it is likely to contain.

Although mostly water, there are several problems with the current crop of mouthwashes. Firstly, most contain alcohol. Use of alcohol-containing mouthwashes is associated with an increased risk of throat and mouth cancers. This is because alcohol is drying, unbalances the pH of the mouth, and strips away the protective mucous membrane in the mouth and throat. Although only in a low concentration, most mouthwashes also contain fluoride. Drinking alcohol- and fluoride-containing mouthwash is a major source of poisoning among young children.

The more claims a mouthwash makes, the more chemicals it is likely to contain.

Breath fresheners – often sprays – are concentrated forms of mouthwash. Typically they contain more alcohol than water as well as *isobutene* (used in cigarette lighters as a fuel), glycerine, sweeteners such as saccharin or sorbitol, flavourings and even colours. Because they are so high in alcohol and they are not rinsed out of the mouth, regular users are at increased risk of throat cancer. Using a spray will not stop you having bad breath.

With good oral hygiene mouthwashes and breath sprays are never necessary. A healthy mouth simply has no odour. If you are experiencing a problem with persistent bad breath it could be because of gum disease or some other underlying infection. This problem is most effectively addressed with a trip to the dentist. Chronic digestive problems can also contribute to bad breath and need to be sorted out through attention to your diet and the presence of potential food allergens.

Dental floss

Although we think of flossing as a recent development in dental care, evidence gleaned from the skulls of prehistoric humans suggests that we have been flossing in one way or another for a very long time. In the 1800s floss was made of fine unwaxed silk thread. Today it is made of thin nylon string.

Some holistic dentists have expressed concern that modern dental floss can be contaminated with mercury-containing antiseptics. Certainly some flosses are impregnated with unnecessary flavourings derived from petrochemicals and some are even coloured. Often they are coated with waxes of petrochemical origin as well.

When buying dental floss, choose one without flavour or colour. Don't over-floss. Being too aggressive with your floss can wear a groove in your teeth and tear your gums, making them more susceptible to infection.

Alternatives for healthy teeth and gums

Remember that it's not the paste but the brush that cleans your teeth. Equally, it's not how hard you brush, but how long and how thoroughly. Brushing hard and fast won't clean your teeth better and it may damage your gums. So instead of just running the brush quickly over your teeth and hoping the toothpaste (or mouthwash) will catch what you don't, consider spending at least a minute (if not two) gently but thoroughly brushing your teeth each morning and night.

UNUSUAL WAYS TO FLOSS

American naturopath Dr Hulda Clark has gone so far as to recommend that flossing is best done with 2- or 4-pound mono filament fishing line (doubled and twisted for strength)! She also suggests that the thin plastic used for most shopping bags is also serviceable. Tear off a thin strip and roll it slightly to make a quick, effective floss.

If you still want to use commercial brands of toothpaste, consider these options:

- **Use less**. In spite of what you see on TV you only need a pea-sized amount of toothpaste (about a quarter of the advertised amount) to clean your teeth. And while children are advised to use a pea-sized amount they can clean their teeth adequately with half this amount, or a 'smear'.
- **Dilute it**. Turn toothpaste into a cream by diluting it with cooled boiled water. Store in a small squeeze top bottle. It will still foam and clean well.
- **Use a low-fluoride toothpaste**. Among brands aimed at adults, a low-fluoride content is around 500ppm. Several children's brands contain even less, and there is nothing (apart from aesthetics) stopping the whole family from using a children's paste to clean their teeth.
- **Buy a fluoride-free brand**, and if you can an *SLS*-free brand. In most large supermarket and chemists it will be almost impossible to find a toothpaste that is fluoride-free and *SLS*-free. Healthfood stores will stock a wider range; but check the labels of 'natural' alternatives for detergents and other dubious chemicals.

Alternatives to conventional toothpastes are not hard to find; they are plentiful in health food shops, by mail order and on the Internet and are beginning to be sold in supermarkets too. Unfortunately, a quick scan of many ingredient labels will show that the so-called alternatives aren't very 'alternative'. In natural toothpastes, chalk or bicarbonate of soda can be substituted for silica and essential oils for *Triclosan,* and glycerine can be used instead of more harmful humectants such as *propylene glycol* but the basic mixture is the same.

Very few toothpastes are free from worrying chemicals of one sort or another. Some contain contentious preservatives such as *parabens*, the potential hormone disrupter used widely in cosmetics. The trick with toothpaste alternatives is to read labels and find one whose basic mix is as natural as possible while still providing the degree of effectiveness, a pleasant feel in the mouth and the taste that you are used to.

SIMPLE ALTERNATIVES

Simple toothpaste can be made from bicarbonate of soda, vegetable glycerine and essential oil of peppermint, lemon or fennel.

As a general rule use 1 part liquid to two parts bicarbonate of soda; thus 50ml (3tbsp) glycerine to 100ml (8tbsp) bicarbonate of soda. You can vary the proportions until you get the consistency you prefer. Add 5 drops of the essential oil of your choice to pep up the flavour. Shake well before use.

This mixture can be stored in a small squeezable or pump dispenser (travel size is ideal), which can be purchased in large chemists. Use sparingly. Don't be tempted to make more than about 50ml at a time. Although the essential oils will act as a preservative, when making your own toiletries it is always safest to make small amounts as needed rather than risk the product going off.

Another way of making this mixture up is to substitute a natural mouthwash – one without alcohol, fluoride, chemical preservatives, flavours or colours – for the glycerine. Mix this with bicarbonate of soda in approximately the same ratio as above.

Simple mouthwash. The simplest mouthwash is a couple of drops of peppermint oil or sage tincture in a cup of water. To make around 100ml (8tbsp) of a more complex blend you need:

- 15 ml (1 tbsp) lavender tincture
- 15 ml (1 tbsp) calendula tincture
- 10ml (2 tsp) aloe juice
- 30 ml (2 tbsp) cooled boiled water
- 30 ml (2 tbsp) vegetable glycerine
- 5 drops peppermint essential oil

Mix the ingredients together and pour them into a bottle. This mixture will keep for up to 6 months. If you have an infection in the mouth or gums substitute echinacea, myrrh or golden seal tinctures for the lavender.

If you feel strongly that you shouldn't put anything in your mouth that you aren't prepared to swallow, then brushing regularly with a tiny amount of baking soda or a few drops of food-grade hydrogen peroxide diluted in water will also clean your teeth adequately. Hydrogen peroxide is a simple germicidal agent composed only of water and oxygen. Most chemists sell a 3 per cent solution of hydrogen peroxide which is safe to use and gives the bonus of gently whitening your teeth.

Bicarbonate of soda is a useful mild abrasive and has antibacterial properties. Since undiluted bicarbonate of soda can be hard on tooth enamel (particularly as you get older and enamel begins to soften) try dissolving a teaspoonful in a little water first and then dipping your toothbrush in the liquid frequently during brushing (do the same when using hydrogen peroxide).

Because bicarbonate of soda doesn't taste great, try making it more palatable by mixing the dry powder in a small, airtight container with a few drops of peppermint oil. Mix well and store for use as and when you need it. You can also make your own toothpaste and mouthwash quite easily.

Chapter 13
A New Perspective

There is always a danger when criticising conventional personal-care products that you will be accused of being too picky and of trying to make people feel guilty about using what is essentially a harmless luxury. When I first started writing about the ingredients in personal-care products, human health was my main focus. The object was to make people aware of what they were putting on their skin and to help them make healthier choices. But today the concern is wider than that because of our knowledge of the environmental effects related to the beauty products we use.

Much of this book is devoted to their impact on human health, as well as how to change behaviour and the perception of what beauty really is. Today, we know that environmentally, these products and the packaging they come in contribute to our dependency on petroleum and cause environmental destruction associated with cutting down forests, mining and refining natural minerals and ores.

You might not think that choosing a natural organic personal-care product is up there with halting climate change or saving the whale, but if you look at our consumer society from a different perspective, you will recognise that everything we buy, use, discard in the bin, flush down the toilet or wash down the drain has an impact on the environment and on the interconnected natural systems that drive our climate.

You will realise that many of our little luxuries aren't harmless, just like the unnecessary trip in the car just to pick up a pint of milk, or the tonnes of completely unnecessary food packaging we throw away each year. Or the gadgets we buy and then toss away when something newer and more amusing comes along.

Believe it or not, there is a clear link between a lipstick or an aerosol deodorant with not just a decline in human health, but a decline in the health of the planet. It doesn't take much foresight to see that when a cosmetic manufacturer uses palm oil in their products they are as guilty as junk-food manufacturers of furthering the destruction of forest habitats of orangutans and tigers. When manufacturers rely on petrochemicals to produce cheap chemicals for beauty products they are as responsible for the depletion of a rapidly declining, non-renewable resource as a major oil company.

Unlike the automotive industry, the chemical industry has within its immediate grasp the means to stop using undesirable ingredients like petrochemicals and be a part of the solution instead of a part of the problem.

As much as many of us might like to, we can't shop to save the world and the best kind of beauty makeover is one where we get back to the basics of good skin and hair care – i.e. a good diet, plenty of water and exercise and enough rest. In terms of personal-care products, most of us need only a few items – soap, shampoo and moisturiser – to keep clean, healthy and beautiful. Many personal-care products, however, promote patterns of excessive consumption through an emphasis on luxury, beauty and physical appearance. Furthermore, a huge percentage of us buy more than we ever use – wasteful behaviour that impacts on our pockets as well as the planet.

Reading through this book, you may have felt dismayed at the overwhelming number of ways in which everyday products can potentially affect your health, as well as have unexpected environmental impacts. But don't give up and don't get discouraged!

Sensible use of cosmetics and toiletries may mean making the occasional compromise. If there is something that you absolutely can't live without, then keep using it. But try to make 'chemical savings' elsewhere in your life by, for instance, saving perfume or make-up for special occasions only, using a fluoride-free toothpaste, cutting down on the number of other largely unnecessary toiletries you use, and trying some of the suggestions in this book for DIY beauty.

You have more power than you think and you can, to a very large and influential extent, learn to pick your poisons and keep your total body load of synthetic chemicals to a minimum. This book gives you an enormous amount of information to help make this process more straightforward. And, as they say, one good thing leads to another. By becoming more discerning about the products you uses, you are doing something positive for your health and for the planet, helping yourself to feel empowered as a consumer, and helping to ensure that you and your family have a healthy future to look forward to.

Select Bibliography

An enormous amount of research has formed the background to this book. These pages represent a selection of the papers and books which readers may find interesting.

Papers and Reports

General

11th Report on Carcinogens, National Toxicology Program, US Department of Health and Human Services, Public Health Service

An Environmental Assessment of alkylphenol ethoxylates and alkylphenols, Warhurst, AM, Friends of the Earth, London, 1995

Biology and Politics: Linking Nature and Nurture, Masters RD, Ann Rev Polit Sci, 2001; 4: 345–69

Exposure to volatile organic compounds in indoor air: A review, Brown SK, Proceedings of the International Clean Air Conference of the Clean Air Society of Australia and New Zealand, 1992; 1: 95-104

Chemical Hazard Data Availability Study: What Do We Really Know About the Safety of High Production Volume Chemicals? EPA, 1998

Crisis in Chemicals: The threat posed by the 'biomedical revolution' to the profits, liabilities and regulation of industries making and using chemicals, Friends of the Earth, May 2000

Dawn of the Domestic Superbug, Thomas P, Ecologist, July/August 2005: 42-8

Draft risk assessment of the potential human health effects associated with exposure to perfluorooctanoic acid and its salts, Environmental Protection Agency, January 4, 2005. Available online at www.epa.gov/oppt/pfoa

Effects of piperonyl butoxide on the toxicity and hepatocarcinogenicity of 2-acetylaminofluorene and 4acetylaminobiphenyl, and their N-hydroxylated derivatives, following administration to newborn mice, Fujii K and Epstein S, Oncol, 1979; 36: 105-12

Environmental and heritable factors in the causation of cancer - Analyses of cohorts of twins from Sweden, Denmark, and Finland, Lichtenstein, P et al, N Eng J Med, 2000; 343: 78-85

Environmental diseases from A to Z. Publication no. 96-4145, National Institutes of Health, US Department of Health and Human Services, 1997

Environmental medicine, Part 1: The human burden of environmental toxins and their common health effects, Crinnion WJ, Altern Med Rev, 2000; 5: 52–63

Everyday exposure to toxic pollutants, Ott WR, Roberts JW, Sci Am, 1998; Feb: 86–91

Health Hazard Information, US Environmental Protection Agency, 1991

How are children different from adults?, Bearer CF, Environmental Health Perspectives, 1995; 103 (Suppl 6): 7–12

How chemical exposures affect reproductive health: Patient fact sheet, Greater Boston Physicians for Social Responsibility, GBPSR, 1996

Human health and chemical mixtures: an overview, Carpenter DO et al, Environmental Health Perspectives, 1998; 106 (Suppl 6):1263-70

Identification of polar organic compounds found in consumer products and their toxicological properties, Cooper SD et al, Anal Environ Epidemiol, 1995; 5: 57-75

Identification of polar volatile organic compounds in consumer products and common microenvironments, US Environmental Protection Agency, 1991

Increasing incidence of non-Hodgkin's lymphoma: occupational and environmental factors, Pearce N and Bethwait P, Cancer Res, 1992; 52(19 Suppl): 5496S-5500S

Introduction to Hormone Disrupting Compounds, Warhurst M. Available online at: http://website.lineone.net/~mwarhurst/

Hormones, and Other Organic Wastewater Contaminants in U.S. Streams, 1999 – 2000: A National Reconnaissance, Kolpin, D et al, Environmental Science and Technology, 2002; 36:1202-11

Effect of antibacterial home cleaning and handwashing products on infectious disease symptoms: a randomized, double-blind trial, Larson EL, Ann Intern Med, 2004; 140 (5): 321-9

Multiple chemical sensitivity recognition and management: A document on the health effects of everyday chemical exposures and their implications, Third scientific report of the British Society for Allergy, Environmental and Nutritional Medicine, Eaton KK and Anthony HM, BSAENM, March 2000

National Report on Human Exposure to Environmental Chemicals, Centers for Disease Control and Prevention, Atlanta, GA: CDC, March 2001; available online at: www.cdc.gov/nceh/dls/report/

Neurogenic inflammation and sensitivity to environmental chemicals, Meggs WJ, Environmental Health Perspectives, 1993; 101: 234-8

Neurogenic switching: A hypothesis for a mechanism for shifting the site of inflammation in allergy and chemicals sensitivity, Meggs WJ, Environmental Health Perspectives, 1995; 103: 54-6

Neurotoxicity resulting from coexposure to pyridostigmine bromide, deet, and permethrin: implications of Gulf War chemical exposures, Abou-Donia MB et al, J Toxicol Environmental Health Perspectives, 1996; 48(1): 35-56

SELECT BIBLIOGRAPHY

Neurotoxins: at home and the workplace, report by the Committee on Science and Technology, US House of Representatives, Sept 15, 1986, No 99-827

Our Stolen Future, Colbin T et al, available online at: www.ourstolenfuture.org

Personal exposure, indoor-outdoor relationships, and breath levels of toxic air pollutants measured for 355 persons in New Jersey. Wallace LA et al, EPA 0589

Personal exposures, outdoor concentrations, and breath levels of toxic air pollutants measured for 425 persons in urban, suburban and rural areas, Wallace LA et al, EPA 0589, presented at the Annual Meeting of Air Pollution Control Association, San Francisco, CA, 25 June 1984

PFCs – A family of chemicals that contaminate the planet, Environmental Working Group, EWG, April 2003

Second national report on human exposure to environmental chemicals, Centers for Disease Control and Prevention, Atlanta, GA, March 2003, available online at: www.cdc.gov/exposurereport/

Solvents and Neurotoxicity, White RF and Proctor SP, Lancet, 1997; 349: 1239–43

Synergistic activation of oestrogen receptors with combinations of environmental chemicals, Arnold SF et al, Science, 1996; 272: 1489-92

The oestrogenic activity of phthalate esters in vitro, Harris C et al, Environmental Health Perspectives, 1997; 105: 802-11

Toxic effects of air freshener emissions, Anderson RC and Anderson JH, Arch Environ Health, 1997; 52: 433–41

Toxic alert. A survey of high street companies and their approach to suspect chemicals, Friends of the Earth, October 2000

Toxic nation: A report on pollution in Canadians, Environmental Defence, Canada Nov 2005 317 Adelaide Street West, Suite 705 Toronto, ON M5V 1P9, see online at: www.environmentaldefence.ca

Volatile organic pollutants in new and established buildings in Melbourne, Australia, Brown SK, Indoor Air, 2002; 12: 55–63

Identification of Polar Volatile Organic Compounds in Consumer Products and Common Microenvironments, Wallace L, EPA, 1991

Toiletries and cosmetics

A case-control study of borderline ovarian tumors: the influence of perineal exposure to talc, Harlow BL and Weiss BS, Am J Epidemiol, 1989; 130: 390-4

A case-control study of hair dye use and breast cancer, Shore RE et al, J Natl Cancer Inst, 1979; 62: 277-83

A prospective study of permanent hair dye use and hematopoietic cancer, Grodstein F et al, J Natl Cancer Inst, 1994; 86: 1466-70

Acute fluoride toxicity from ingesting home-use dental products in children, birth to 6 years of age, Shulman JD and Wells LM, J Publ Health Dent, 1997; 57: 150–8

Acute toxic effects of fragrance products, Anderson RC and Anderson JH, Arch Environ Health, 1998; 53: 138–46

Concentrations of parabens in human breast tumours, Darbre PD, et al, J Appl Toxicol. 2004 Jan–Feb;24(1): 5–13

Fluoride in dental products: safety considerations, Whitford GM, J Dent Res, 1987; 66, 1056-1060

Fragrance compounds and essential oils with sedative effects upon inhalation, Buchbauer G et al, J Pharm Sci, 1993; 82: 660-4

Genital talc exposure and risk of ovarian cancer, Cramer DW et al, Int J Cancer, 1999; 81: 351-6

Hair dye use and multiple myeloma in white men, Brown LM et al, Am J Public Health, 1992; 82: 1673-4

Hair dye use and risk of fatal cancers in US women, Thun MJ et al, J Natl Cancer Inst, 1994; 86: 210-5

Hair dye use and risk of leukaemia and lymphoma, Cantor KP et al, Am J Publ Health, 1988; 78: 570-1

Hair product use and the risk of breast cancer in young women, Cook LS et al, Cancer Causes Control, 1999; 10: 551-9

Hair-color products and risk for non-Hodgkin's lymphoma: a population-based study in the San Francisco bay area, Holly EA et al, Am J Publ Health, 1998; 88: 1767-73

Have you met this syndrome?, Lawson R, Medical Monitor, September 4, 1996: 66

In vitro and in vivo estrogenicity of UV screens, Schlumpf M et al, Environmental Health Perspectives, 2001; 109: 239-44

Inhalation challenge effects of perfume scent strips in patients with asthma, Kumar P et al, Ann Allergy Asthma Immunol, 1995; 75: 429-33

Mutagenicity of cosmetic products containing Kathon, Connor TH et al, Environ Mol Mutagen, 1996; 28: 127-32

Neurotoxic fragrance produces ceroid and myelin disease, Spencer PS et al, Science, 1979; 204: 633-5

Neurotoxic properties of musk ambrette, Spencer PS et al, Toxicol Appl Pharmacol, 1984; 75: 571-5

N-Nitrosoalkanolamines in cosmetics in relevance to human cancer of N-nitroso compounds, tobacco smoke and mycotoxins, Eisenbrand G, et al IARC 1991

Occurrence of nitro and non-nitro benzenoid musk compounds in human adipose tissue, Mauller S et al Chemosphere, 1996; 33: 17-28

Olfactory primary neurons as a route of entry for toxic agents into the CNS, Hastings L et al, Neurotoxicology, 1991; 12: 707-14

Patch testing with fragrances: results of a multicentre of the European environmental and contact dermatitis research group with 48 frequently used constituents of perfumes, Frosch PJ et al, Contact Dermatitis, 1995; 33: 333-42

Penetration of the fragrance compounds, cinnamaldehyde and cinnamyl alcohol, through human skin in vitro, Weibel H et al, Contact Dermatitis, 1996; 34: 423-6

Pharmaceuticals and personal-care products in the environment: agents of subtle change, Daughton C and Ternes T, Environmental Health Perspectives, 1999; 107(suppl 6): 907-38

Pharmaceuticals and personal-care products in the environment: agents of subtle change?, Daughton CG and Ternes TA, Environmental Health Perspectives, 1999; 107 (Suppl 6): 907-38

Placebo-controlled challenges with perfume in patients with asthma-like symptoms, Millqvist E and Lowhagen O, Allergy, 1996; 51: 434-9

Potential of carcinogenic effects of hair dyes, Shafer N and Shafer RW, NY State J of Med, 1976; 76: 394-6

Prospective study of talc use and ovarian cancer, Gertig DM et al, J Natl Cancer Inst, 2000; 92: 249-52

Relationship of hair dye use, benign breast disease, and breast cancer, Nasca PC et al, J Natl Cancer Inst, 1980; 64: 23-8

Some alkyl hydroxy benzoate preservatives (parabens) are oestrogenic, Routledge EJ et al, Toxicol Applied Pharmacol, 1998; 153: 12-19

The association between aluminum-containing products and Alzheimer's disease, Graves AB et al, J Clin Epidemiol, 1990; 43: 35-44

The relationship between perineal cosmetic talc usage and ovarian talc particle burden, Heller DS et al, Am J Obstet Gynecol, 1996; 74: 1507-10

Books

1001 Chemicals in Everyday Products, 2nd ed, Ross Lewis G, Wiley-Interscience, 1999

Chemical Exposures: Low Levels and High Stakes, Ashford N and Miller C, Wiley & Sons, 1998

Chemistry and Biology of N-nitroso Compounds, Lijinsky W, Cambridge University Press, 1990

Cleaning Yourself to Death, Thomas P, New Leaf, 2001

Clinical Toxicology of Commercial Products, 5th ed, Gosselin RE et al, Williamson & Wilkins, 1984

Cosmetics Unmasked, Antczak Dr S and G, Thorsons, 2001

Enquire Within, 3rd ed, Bremner M, Helicon, 1994

Feeding Your Skin, Oates C, Vermilion, 2007

Living Dangerously, Thomas P, New Leaf, 2003

Living Healthy in a Toxic World, Steinman D and Wisner RM, Perigree, 1996

Make Your Own Cosmetics, Neal's Yard Remedies, Aurum Press, 1997

Overview of similarities and differences between children and adults: implications for risk assessment, Roberts RJ, in Guzelian PS et al, (eds), Similarities and Differences Between Children and Adults. Washington, DC: ILSI Press, 1992: 1–15

Secret Ingredients, Cox P and Brusseau P, Bantam Books, 1997

The Breast Cancer Prevention Program, Epstein S et al, Macmillan, 1997

The Complete Guide to Household Chemicals, Palma RJ, Prometheus Books, 1995

The Fragrant Pharmacy, Wormwood VA, Macmillan, 1990

The Precautionary Principle in Action – A Handbook, Tickner J et al, Science and Environmental Health Network, 1998

The Safe Shopper's Bible – A Consumer's Guide to Nontoxic Household Products, Steinman D and Epstein S, Macmillan, 1995

The Top 100 Traditional Remedies, Merson S, Duncan Baird, 2006

Unreasonable Risk, Epstein S, Environmental Toxicology, Inc, 2001

What's In This Stuff?, Thomas P, Rodale, 2006

Whole Foods Companion, Onstad D, Chelsea Green, 1996

You Are What You Eat, McKeith G, Michael Joseph, 2004

Appendix 1

Cancer
Concerns

Most of us are aware of the allergenic potential of cosmetics and toiletries and that manufacturers work hard to reduce the short-term irritation factor of ingredients such as preservatives and fragrances. But what may come as a shock is that there are longer-term risks associated with continual use of cosmetics and toiletries. Many, for instance, contain known carcinogens.

Manufacturers argue that these ingredients are only present in tiny amounts and so could not possibly be harmful, but without long-term research – which manufacturers have shown themselves unwilling to fund – the possibility that cosmetic use could lead to cancer is difficult to prove. Nevertheless, some types of cosmetics such as hair dyes are already being linked with higher rates of specific cancers among users (see Chapter 10).

According to Dr Samuel Epstein, Chairman of the Cancer Prevention Coalition, there are two classes of major carcinogenic ingredients in cosmetics and toiletries.

The first class includes those ingredients that are carcinogenic. These are known as 'frank' carcinogens. The second group are known as 'hidden' or co-carcinogens. These chemicals, while not carcinogenic themselves, may under certain conditions develop carcinogenic properties – for instance when mixed together – or increase the carcinogenic potential of other chemicals. More than 40 frank carcinogens and more than 30 hidden carcinogens are commonly used in everyday personal-care products – including those intended for children.

Frank carcinogens

The list of frank carcinogens is comprised mostly of synthetic coal-tar dyes commonly used to colour cosmetics and hair dyes, as well as solvents and preservatives that can be found on almost every cosmetic label. As an eye-opening exercise, check for yourself if your favourite products contain any of these ingredients:

- *Benzyl acetate*
- *Butyl benzylphthalate*
- *Butylated hydroxyanisole (BHA)*
- *Butylated hyroxytoluene (BHT)*
- Crystalline silica
- D&C green 5 (CI61570)
- D&C orange 17 (CI12075)
- D&C red 2, 3, 4, 10, 17★
- D&C red 8, 9,19 and 33 (CI15585/CI45170/CI17200)
- *Diaminophenol*
- *Diethanolamine (DEA)*
- *Dioctyl adipate*
- Disperse blue 1 (CI64500)
- Disperse yellow 3 (CI11855)
- Ethyl alcohol
- FD & C blue 1 and 2 (CI42090/CI73015)
- FD&C blue 4★
- FD & C green 3 (CI42053)
- FD & C red 4, and 40 (CI14700/CCI16035)
- FD&C red 10★
- FD & C yellow 5 and 6 (CI19140/CI15985)
- Fluoride
- Formaldehyde
- *Glutaral*
- *Hydroquinone*
- *Methylene chloride*
- *Nitrophenylenediamine*
- *Phenyl-p-phenylenediamine*
- *Polyvinylpyrrolidone*
- *p-phenylenediamine*
- *Pyrocatechol*
- Saccharin
- Talc
- *Titanium dioxide*

★ Now banned from cosmetics in the US and Europe

Hidden carcinogens

In general, hidden carcinogens can be broken down into three main categories: formaldehyde-releasers, nitrosamine-precursors and contaminants. Formaldehyde-releasers and nitrosamine-precursors are generally preservatives, solvents, carriers and detergents/surfactants. These are always listed on the label.

Formaldehyde is a skin irritant and known carcinogen, so products with these ingredients on their own carry a certain amount of risk. But when formaldehyde-releasers and nitrosamine-precursors are mixed in the same formula they can produce potent cancer-causing agents called nitrosamines. Studies show that between 42 and 93 per cent of toiletries and cosmetics contain these compounds, which are quickly and easily absorbed into the skin from both leave-on and wash-off products. Again, check the labels of your favourite cosmetics for these formaldehyde-releasing substances:

- *2-bromo-2-nitropropane-1,3-diol (Bronopol)*
- *Diazolidinyl urea*
- *DMDM hydantoin*
- *Imidazolidinyl urea*
- *Metheneamine*
- *Quarternium-15*
- *Sodium/Hydroxymethylglycinate*

Nitrosamine-precursors are among the most dangerous chemicals we put in and on our bodies in the name of beauty. They belong to a family of hormone-disrupting chemicals and are almost always found in products that foam, such as bubble bath, body washes, shampoos, liquid soaps and facial cleansers. Some of the most common of these ingredients are:

- *Bromonitrodioxane*
- *Bronopol* (aka *2-bromo-2-nitropropane-1,3-diol*)
- Cocamide DEA
- Cocamide MEA
- *DEA olet-3 phosphate*
- *DEA-cetyl phosphate*
- *Diethanolamine (DEA)*
- *Lauramide DEA*
- *Linoleamide MEA*
- *Metheneamine*
- *Monethanolamine*
- *Morpholine*
- *Myristamide DEA*
- *Oleamide DEA*
- *Padimate-O* (aka *octyldimethyl para-amino benzoic acid*)
- *Pyroglutamic acid*
- *Stearalkonium chloride*
- *Stearamide MEA*
- *TEA lauryl sulfate*
- *TEA-Sodium Lauryl Sulphate*
- *Triethanolamine (TEA)*

Once added to the product, these chemicals readily react with any nitrites present to form the carcinogenic nitrosamine *NDELA* (*N-nitrosodiethanolamine*). Nitrosamines are one of the major carcinogens in cigarettes and are also found in cured meats. In the 1970s nitrosamine contamination of bacon and other cured meats became a worldwide public health issue. The nitrosamine content of cured meats has dropped drastically in recent years. However, the nitrosamine content of toiletries is alarmingly high. In a single shampoo you could absorb 50–100 micrograms of nitrosamine through the skin. To put this in perspective, a typical portion of bacon would only supply 1 microgram of nitrosamine.

Nitrites can get into personal-care products in several ways. They can be added as anti-corrosive agents and be present as contaminants in raw materials. They can also be the result of the presence of formaldehyde-releasing chemicals in the mix.

The long shelf life of most toiletries increases the risk of carcinogenic chemical reaction. Stored for extended periods at elevated temperatures, nitrates will continue to form in a product, accelerated by the presence of certain other chemicals such as formaldehyde, *paraformaldehyde*, *thiocyanate*, *nitrophenols* and certain metal salts.

Inadequate and confusing labelling means that consumers may never know which products are most likely to be contaminated. However, a 1980 FDA report stated that approximately 42 per cent of all cosmetics were contaminated with *NDELA* – shampoos having the highest concentrations. In two 1991 reports, 27 out of 29 products tested were found to be contaminated with *NDELA*.

While manufacturers plead that *DEA* and its relatives are safe in products that are designed for brief or discontinuous use, or those which wash off, there is evidence from both human and animal studies that *DEA* is quickly absorbed through the skin. This argument does not explain why these chemicals crop up regularly in body lotions and facial moisturisers, which are not washed off.

As far back as 1978, the International Agency for Research on Cancer (IARC) concluded that *N-nitrosodiethanolamine* should be regarded for practical purposes as if it were carcinogenic to humans. The IARC maintain this position on *NDELA* today.

In 1994 in the US the National Toxicology Program similarly concluded that, 'There is sufficient evidence for the carcinogenicity of *N-nitrodiethanolamine* in experimental animals.' It noted that of over 44 different species in which *NDELA* compounds have been tested, all have been susceptible, and that humans were most unlikely to be the only exception to this trend.

Worryingly, the response of the cosmetic industry to the problem of nitrosamiane-formation in their products has been to put even more chemicals, such as preservatives and antioxidants, in their products in an attempt to slow or inhibit the formation on *NDELA*. None have been proved adequate against all possible nitrosating agents found in everyday cosmetics.

Contaminants

Carcinogens can get into your toiletries in other ways. Contaminants end up in cosmetics due to careless processing of the starting materials and as such are not listed on the label:

- *Aflatoxin* – in peanut oil and flour
- *Arsenic* – in coal tar dyes, polyvinyl acetate, *PEG (polyethylene glycols)* compounds
- *Chloroaniline* – in chlorhexidine
- *Crystalline silica* – in amorphous (powdered) silicates used in toothpastes and make-up
- **DDT, Dieldrin, Endrin and other organochlorine pesticides** – in lanolin, hydrogenated cottonseed oil, *quarternium-26*
- **DEA (diethanolamine)** – in *DEA-cocamide/lauramide* condensates, *quarternium-26*
- **1,4-Dioxane** – in ethoxylated alcohols, including *PEGs, polysorbate 60 & 80, nonoxynol* and chemicals with 'eth' in the name (e.g. *choleth-24, ceteareth-3, laureths*)
- *Ethylhexylacrylate* – in acrylate and methacrylate polymers
- *Ethylene oxide* – in *PEGs, oleths, ceteareth-3, laureths, polysorbate 60 & 80, nonoxynol*
- **Formaldehyde** – in *polyoxymethylene urea*
- **Lead** – in coal-tar dyes, *polyvinyl acetate, PEG-(polyethylene glycols)* compounds

In addition to these, many of today's toiletries are based on compounds called ethoxylated alcohols. Ethoxylates can be contaminated with the carcinogen *1,4-dioxane*. Commonly used ethoxylates include *PEG, polyethylene, polyethylene glycol, polyoxyethylene*, 'eth' compounds such as *sodium laureth sulfate* or *oxynol. Polysorbate 60* and *Polysorbate 80* may also contain this contaminant.

In one 1991 study of a range of products including shampoos, liquid soaps, suncreams, bath foams, moisturising lotions, aftershave balms, cleansing milks, baby lotions, facial creams and hair lotions, more than half the products contained dioxanes at levels potentially harmful to human health.

Appendix 2
Chemicals A–Z

The number of chemicals we encounter each day is staggering and it would take several full volumes just to list them all. However, some chemicals turn up in our personal-care products more frequently than others and this A–Z provides snapshot of their potential effects. A little background information may help you understand the information in this section. First of all, chemicals can be absorbed into the body in several ways, for instance:

- through the respiratory tract via inhalation
- through the skin via dermal contact
- through the digestive tract via ingestion (Ingestion can occur if a chemical is present in products that are applied to the mouth or through transfer from hands or food, for example)

A chemical may have serious effects by one route of exposure and minimal effects by another. It can also be relatively safe in small or dilute concentrations but show serious adverse effects as the concentration goes up.

In addition, chemicals can produce both local and systemic effects. With a local effect the chemicals does not need to be absorbed to produce an effect. Instead it takes place at the point or area of contact. The site can be skin, mucous membranes, the respiratory tract, gastrointestinal system or the eyes. Such chemicals are known as irritants because they can cause inflammation of the skin and the mucous membranes in the eyes, nose or respiratory system.

A systemic effect refers to an adverse health effect that takes place at a location distant from the body's initial point of contact with the chemical caused by the chemical being absorbed into the body. Substances with systemic effects often have 'target organs' in which they accumulate and exert their toxic effect such as the kidneys, liver or heart. Some substances that cause systemic effects are cumulative poisons. These substances tend to build up in the body as a result of numerous chronic exposures, which is why it is important to try and make long-term changes to your beauty regime.

Chemicals that cause systemic effects can further be classified as:

- **Reproductive toxins**. Cause impotence or sterility in men and women.
- **Carcinogens**. Substances that can cause cancer.
- **Mutagens**. Anything that causes a change in the genetic material of a living cell. Many mutagens are also carcinogens.
- **Teratogens** A substance that interferes with the developing embryo and can cause birth defects when a pregnant woman is exposed to that substance.
- **Neurotoxins**. Affect the nervous system. Some diseases associated with nervous system damage include multiple sclerosis, Parkinson's disease, Alzheimer's disease and sudden infant death syndrome.

When exposure occurs to several substances simultaneously the resultant systemic toxic effect may be significantly greater in combination than the additive toxic effect of each substance alone. This is called a synergistic effect. Good examples of this include simultaneous exposure to alcohol and chlorinated solvents, or to cigarette smoke and asbestos.

Not everyone will experience the reactions listed here. Indeed, that is the frustrating thing about chemical research. We know so little about who is likely to react, and why and to what extent. For this reason this A–Z tries to be as compressive as possible about known adverse reactions.

2-BROMO-2-NITROPROPANE-1,3-DIOL
Bronopol
Preservative found in toiletries, cosmetics and household cleaners. It is a formaldehyde-forming chemical (formaldehyde is a carcinogen) which can react with nitrosating ingredients in the mix to form carcinogenic nitrosamines (see Appendix 1 for more).

2-NITRO-p-PHENYLENEDIAMINE
See *Phenylenediamines*

4-AMINO-2-NITROPHENOL
p-Aminonitrophenol
Used as an oxidising agent in permanent and semi-permanent hair dyes. Linked to bladder cancer in animal and human studies.

4-CHLORO-m-PHENYLENEDIAMINE
See *Phenylenediamines*

144

ACETAMIDE MEA

N- 2- hydroxyethylacetamide

A humectant (wetting agent) used in cosmetics such as lipsticks and cream blushers to retain moisture. In the short-term, *acetamide* can cause mild skin irritation. Chronic ingestion has produced benign and malignant liver tumours in rats and an increased incidence of malignant lymphomas in mice. May be contaminated with harmful impurities linked to cancer and other health disorders (see *Monoethanolamine*).

ACETONE

Dimethyl Ketone, Methyl Ketone

An industrial denaturant and solvent used in the manufacture of premoistened towelettes, nail polish remover and perfumes. Also used in some skin-cleaning formulas for its ability to dissolve fats and grease. Used on the skin it can produce skin rashes, dryness and irritation. Inhalation even for short periods can provoke nose, throat, lung and eye irritation, headaches, light-headedness and fatigue. Chronic exposure can damage the kidneys and liver.

ACRYLATES

Film formers, emulsifiers and surfactants that help the cosmetics and body-care products stick to the skin and can make it feel softer. Their safety has not been thoroughly investigated. Although they are presumed non-toxic, they can be skin and eye irritants.

ALCOHOL, DENATURED

Ethanol, Ethyl alcohol

A solvent used extensively in the manufacture of varnishes, artificial flavourings, perfumes and inks. It's clear and colourless and highly inflammable. Used on the skin it can cause dryness and irritation over time. Ingestion of small amounts can cause behavioural changes and impairment of vision; large amounts can cause nausea, vomiting, coma and death.

ALKYL COMPOUNDS

Alkyl compounds are used as surfactants and detergents found in cosmetics, toiletries, household goods and pesticides. They are problematic in many ways. One common type, the alkyl *benzyl sulfonates* (*ABS*) group, includes *linear alkyl benzene sulfonates* (*LAS*) and *linear alkyl sodium sulfonates* both of which are slow to biodegrade. *LAS* are the most common surfactants in use in household products.

ALKYLPHENOLS

Nonylphenol, Nonylphenoxy ethoxylates, Alkylphenol polyglycol, Poylethylene glycol alkyl aryl ethers

Surfactants and detergents found in household cleaners, laundry detergents, cosmetics, pesticides, paints and varnishes. *Alkylphenols* are still used in commercial products in the US, but are confined to industrial detergents in the UK. They can easily get into the water supply and food chain and are hormone disrupters believed to be contributing to reproductive problems in men such as low sperm counts, damaged sperm and testicular cancer. Many *alkylphenols* are toxic to aquatic organisms and are implicated in the feminisation of male fish.

Alkylphenols are hormone disrupters. One member of this family of chemicals is the spermicide *nonoxynyl* (used on condoms and in spermicidal foams and gels), which may give some idea of their powerful biological toxicity.

ALPHA HYDROXY ACIDS

Alpha hydroxy acids or *AHAs* come from a variety of sources including citrus fruits such as grapefruit and papaya. Lactic acid is an *AHA*. In their more concentrated form *AHAs* are used by dermatologists to remove the top layers of the skin, usually as a treatment for skin diseases and wrinkles. While not in skin products at anywhere near this concentration, the effect of *AHAs* is still to burn the skin slightly. The 'glow' you get from products containing *AHAs* is actually a mild irritation caused by the chemical burn. Some people react more violently to this burning than others and AHAs are reported to be a major cause of adverse reactions to soaps, shampoos and moisturisers.

ALUM

Potassium alum

Usually refers to synthetic aluminium-containing crystals produced in the lab for commercial use as natural deodorants. A powdered form of alum is used as an astringent to prevent bleeding from small shaving cuts. The styptic pencils sold for this purpose contain *aluminium sulfate* or *potassium aluminium sulfate*. Similar products are also used on animals to prevent bleeding after nail-clipping.

ALUMINA

Aluminium oxide

See *Aluminium*

ALUMINUM

One of the most abundant minerals on the planet, aluminium has many uses in household products. It is a colour additive in cosmetics (especially eye shadows) and in foods. It is also a common ingredient in antacids and used in deodorants and antiperspirants (most commonly as *aluminium chlorhydrate, aluminium zirconium, aluminium chloride, alumina, aluminium sulphate* and *aluminium phenosulphate*).

The human body has no dietary requirement for aluminium and ingesting large doses is considered toxic, carcinogenic and mutagenic. Applied to the skin (for instance in deodorants) it is an irritant and with a lifetime's use has been associated with an increased risk of developing Alzheimer's disease. Products containing *aluminium zirconium* compounds have been shown to cause granulomas (small nodules of chronically inflamed tissue) under the arms with prolonged use.

ALUMINIUM CHLOROHYDRATE

See *Aluminium*

ALUMINIUM PHENOSULPHATE
See *Aluminium*

ALUMINIUM SULPHATE
See *Aluminium*

ALUMINUM ZIRCONIUM TETRACHLOROHYDREX GLY
See *Aluminium*

AMINOMETHYL PROPANOL
2-amino-2-methylpropanol

A thickener and gelling agent used in cosmetics. It is a skin irritant which can be contaminated with harmful impurities. As an amine it can mix with other chemicals in the product to form carcinogenic nitrosamine compounds, on the skin or in the body after absorption (see Appendix 1 for more).

AMMONIUM LAURETH SULPHATE

Surfactant found in shampoos and foaming bath products. Although considered mild, it can be irritating to sensitive skin. *Laureth* compounds can be contaminated with *1,4-dioxane* a known carcinogen. Since consumers have no way of knowing which *laureth* compounds are contaminated, avoidance is the safest option.

AMMONIUM LAURYL SULPHATE
Ammonium dodecyl sulphate

Surfactant found in shampoos and foaming bath products. It can be mildly irritating to the skin.

A-TERPINEOL
Alpha terpineol

Synthetic fragrance found in perfume, cologne, laundry detergent, fabric softeners and air fresheners, perfumes, aftershaves, hairsprays and deodorants. Highly irritating to mucous membranes. Inhalation can cause excitement, loss of muscular coordination, hypothermia, central nervous system and respiratory depression and headache.

AVOBENZONE
Butyl methoxy-dibenzoylmethane

Broad spectrum synthetic sunscreen ingredient that can protect against the entire range of the sun's UVA rays. Studies suggest that it is a potential hormone disrupter.

AZO DYES

A large category of dyes used in foods and cosmetics as well as for dyeing textile such as cotton, silk, wool, viscose and synthetic fibres. They are considered to be easy to use, relatively cheap and to provide clear, strong colours. There are approximately 2,000 azo dyes on the market.

The majority of azo dyes are water-soluble and are, therefore, easy for the body to absorb. Absorption takes place through inhalation and swallowing of dust as well as through skin contact. In humans, azo dyes can cause allergic reactions including hives. Many are considered neurotoxic and carcinogenic. Azo dyes can cause 'cross reactivity' with the *phenylenediamine* colourants used in hair dyes. This means that if you are sensitive to one type of dye you can, over time, develop a sensitivity to the other. Azo dyes, which frequently get washed down the drain, may also be toxic to aquatic organisms and cause long-term damage to aquatic environments.

BENZALDEHYDE

Various *benzaldehyde* compounds are used as synthetic fragrances. *Benzaldehyde, 4-methoxy-* for instance, is a sharp bitter almond/cherry fragrance, while *benzaldehyde, 4-hydroxy-3-methoxy* (or *Vanillan*) has a vanilla fragrance. *Benzaldehydes* can be irritating to the mouth, throat, eyes, skin, lungs and gastrointestinal tract, causing nausea and abdominal pain. They have been linked to kidney damage, cellular mutations and central nervous system disruption and in the lab.

BENZALKONIUM CHLORIDE

Alkyl benzyl dimethylammonium chloride

A Quaternary Ammonium Compound used typically as a disinfectant and preservative. Found in disinfecting hand soaps, mouthwashes and aftershave preparations, as well as dishwashing detergent, disinfectants and cleaners, it can be a severe irritant to the eyes and skin if used in high concentrations. Its wide use is causing new strains of resistant bacteria. Laboratory studies suggest it may cause reproductive defects and act as a mutagen.

BENZENE

A carcinogenic solvent derived from petroleum. Found in lacquers, varnishes, oven cleaners, detergents, furniture polish, air fresheners, spot removers, nail polish remover and perfumes. Irritating to mucous membranes and poisonous when ingested.

Harmful amounts may be absorbed through the skin through the use of everyday products and may cause sensitivity to light as well as produce skin rashes and swelling. Benzene is a carcinogen and also a powerful bone marrow poison, destroying the bone marrow's ability to produce blood cells.

BENZOIC ACID

Carboxybenzene

Food and cosmetic preservative and member of the larger family of *benzoates*, used to inhibit the growth of mould, yeast and some bacteria. Also used as a pesticide. Although it occurs naturally in many plants, most commercial benzoic acid is synthetic. People who suffer from asthma, rhinitis or hives (urticaria) may find their symptoms get worse after consuming benzoates.

BENZOPHENONES

Used as fixatives in perfumes. Some *benzophenones* such as *Dioxybenzone, Oxybenzone, Sulisobenzone* and *Benzphenone-3* absorb ultra-violet light and are therefore used as a sunscreen agent, especially for UVA protection. In sensitive individuals they can provoke allergic reactions and photosensitivity.

BENZOYL PEROXIDE

Found in products to treat acne, *benzoyl peroxide* loosens and removes the top layer of skin and kills bacteria on the skin. Can cause contact dermatitis and sensitisation. Not to be used in cases of Acne rosacea. Animal studies suggest that used topically it can promote the formation of skin tumours in animals.

BENZYL ACETATE

Synthetic fragrance with a floral, fruity aroma. Its vapours are irritating to eyes and respiratory passages and may cause coughing. It can be absorbed through the skin causing systemic effects. Long-term use has been linked to pancreatic cancer.

BENZYL ALCOHOL

Benzenemethanol

Solvent and synthetic fragrance found in a wide variety of fragranced household products including perfumes and air fresheners and as well as foods. Applied topically it is irritating to skin and mucous membranes Inhaled it is irritating to the upper respiratory tract and can cause headache, nausea, vomiting, dizziness, drop in blood pressure, central nervous system depression and, in rare cases, death due to respiratory failure. Potential carcinogen.

BENZYL CINNAMATE

See *Cinnamates*

BENZYL SALICYLATE

See *Salicylates*

BETA HYDROXY ACIDS

BHAs

Can be derived from many natural sources. *BHAs* like salicylic acid are often found in anti-ageing creams and other types of cosmetics where they are used to burn off the top layers of skin. *BHAs* are similar to *Alpha hydroxy acids* but are considered marginally less irritating to the skin.

BRONOPOL

See *2-bromo-2-nitropropane-1,3-diol*

BUTANE

Common propellant. Chronic exposure can produce a range of central nervous system symptoms such as headache, breathing difficulties, mood swings, nausea, vomiting, dizziness and symptoms mimicking drunkenness. Butane is a highly inflammable volatile organic chemical (VOC) popular with solvent abusers because it produce a quick 'high'. However, it can also produce convulsions, coma and a quick death. VOCs accumulate in human breast milk. While butane doesn't destroy the earth's ozone layer, it does contribute to the formation of ground-level ozone, or smog, which can cause serious breathing problems. See also *isobutane* and *propane*.

BUTYLATED HYDROXYTOLUENE
BHT
Although commonly used in toiletries and pre-packaged foods, *BHT* is most widely used as an antioxidant in rubber and plastic and in liquid petroleum products such as gasoline and motor oil. Exposure through the skin or through ingestion can trigger contact allergies and dermatitis. Some evidence suggests *BHT* is a potential carcinogen and reproductive toxin. Once in the bloodstream, *BHT* can accelerate the breakdown of Vitamin D (necessary to maintain immunity and healthy bones and teeth).

BUTYLENE GLYCOL
Used in cosmetics as an humectant, solvent and fragrance fixative (keeps the scent strong). It can also be used as a preservative. Has a similar toxicity as Ethylene glycol, which when ingested may cause depression, vomiting, drowsiness, coma, respiratory failure, convulsions, renal damage, kidney failure and death. It is a formaldehyde former and penetration enhancer.

BUTYLPARABEN
See *Parabens*

C13-14 ISOPARAFFIN
A solvent and lubricating agent derived from petrochemicals. It is a relative of mineral oil used to make the product go on smoothly, but may cause skin irritation and increase photosensitivity of the skin.

CALCIUM THIOGLYCOLATE
Calcium mercaptoacetate
Depilatory (hair removing) chemical that has never been fully assessed for safety by any relevant group or association.

CAPRYLIC/CAPRIC TRIGLYCERIDE
Fractionated coconut oil
Emollient and solvent derived from plants, vegetable oils and dairy fats. Commonly used in soaps and skincare formulas. It is also sometimes used as synthetic flavouring in foods. No known safety concerns.

CARBOMER

A gelling agent. It is a synthetic polymer (a plastic-like material) used to thicken, stabilise and promote the shelf life of cosmetic products. No adverse effects known, though this substance is poorly studied.

CARBOXYMETHYLCELLULOSE

A synthetic gum used in creams and lotions as an emulsifier and stabilizer. It has been shown to cause cancer in animals when ingested. Its toxicity in topical applications is unknown.

CETEARYL ALCOHOL

Cetyl stearyl alcohol, emulsifying wax

Emollient, moisturiser, emulsifier that can be animal, vegetable or petrochemical in origin. It closely resembles human sebum (the waxy substance that protects the skin) Largely non-toxic though in sensitive individuals it can cause contact dermatitis, hives and skin sensitisation.

CHLOROBENZENE

Benzene chloride, Chlorobenzol

A solvent used in dyes, pesticides and perfumes, also used for degreasing automobile parts. Harmful if swallowed, inhaled or absorbed through skin. In the short term it is a skin irritant; over the longer term it is considered a possible carcinogen.

CHLOROFLUOROCARBONS

CFCs

Aerosol propellants such as *trichloromethane* and *dichlorodifluoromethane* used to disperse cleaning solvents and degreasers, paints, pesticides and cosmetics. Once in the atmosphere CFCs stay there for a long time (several decades) and are the main cause of stratospheric ozone depletion and therefore important contributors to the phenomenon of global warming.

CHLORHEXIDINE

An antimicrobial used in mouthwashes, sprays and dental gels to prevent and treat the redness, swelling and bleeding gums associated with gingivitis. It is considered effective but with regular use can discolour teeth and is implicated in rising rates of resistant bacteria.

CINNAMATES

A family of sunscreen agents that include *octocrylene, octyl methoxycinnamate* and *cinoxate. Cinnamates* are derivatives of cinnamon and are chemically related to balsam of Peru, tolu balsam, coca leaves, *cinnamic aldehyde* and *cinnamic oil.* People with sensitivities to these chemicals may get an allergic reaction to sunscreens containing *cinnamates.* The *cinnamates* are much less potent than many other chemicals sunscreens and require the addition of other UVB absorbers to achieve higher SPFs. Laboratory studies suggest some *cinnamates* may act like oestrogens in the body.

CINNAMYL ALCOHOL

Synthetic fragrance with a sweet, balsam, hyacinth odour. It is a common skin and eye irritant.

CINOXATE

See *Cinamates*

CITRAL

Synthetic lemon fragrance used in perfumes, household cleaners and air fresheners and in foods. Citral is an allergen and irritant; it has oestrogenic effects and has been found to cause enlargement of the prostate gland in animals.

CITRIC ACID

Food acid, naturally derived from citrus fruit, used in foods and cosmetics. In cosmetics it is a preservative and also an *alpha hyroxy acid*, used to strip the top layers of the skin (supposedly revealing 'younger' skin underneath). Like all *AHAs*, citric acid can cause irritation. As *AHAs* become more popular in cosmetics like soaps, shampoos and moisturisers, they have also become a major cause of adverse skin reactions.

CITRONELLOL

Synthetic fragrance and flavouring. In perfumes it provides a sweet, rose-like odour. Also used as a pesticide to combat mosquitoes and other flying insects. Applied topically it can be a severe skin irritant.

COAL TAR

The black residue obtained by the distillation of coal. Often found in anti-dandruff treatments and in products used to treat seborrheic dermatitis and psoriasis. Can be found in some bath soaps. It may cause photosensitivity in some and with prolonged use also make itching worse. The American Environmental Protection Agency (EPA) classifies coal tar as a human carcinogen.

COCAMIDE DEA

Cocamide diethanolamine
Found in dishwashing liquids, shampoos and cosmetics, *cocamide DEA* is a strong detergent, foam stabiliser and thickener. It can irritate the skin. It also belongs to a family of fatty acids called *alkanolamines*, which are considered hormone-disrupting chemicals. While not carcinogenic on its own, it has the potential to form carcinogenic nitrosamines when mixed with formaldehyde-forming ingredients (see Appendix 1 for more).

COCAMIDE MEA
See *Cocamide DEA*

COCAMIDOPROPYL BETAINE
A detergent that is a strong allergen and skin and eye irritant. It is also a penetration enhancer – allowing other chemicals in the mix to be more easily absorbed through the skin. Can be contaminated with *diethanolamine (DEA)*, which when combined with formaldehyde (released by other ingredients during storage) produces carcinogenic nitrosamines (see Appendix 1 for more).

CYCLOHEXASILOXANE
See *Silicones*

CYCLOMETHICONE
See *Silicones*

CYCLOPENTASILOXANE
See *Silicones*

D-LIMONENE
See *Limonene*

DEA-OLETH-3 PHOSPHATE
Surfactant found in cosmetics and toiletries. A relative of *polyethylene glycol (PEG)*. It can be carcinogenic in itself as well as being contaminated with the carcinogen *1,4-dioxane* (see also *diethanolamine*).

DEA CETYL PHOSPHATE
See *Diethanolamine*

DIAMINOPHENOL
Oxidizing colouring agents in general hair-dyeing products. Can cause allergic reaction and should never be used to dye eyelashes or eyebrows.

DIAMINOTOLUENES
Intermediates in the synthesis of dyes used for textiles, furs, leathers, spirit varnishes and wood stains and pigments. Once widely used in hair-dyes, *2,4-diamontoluene* was removed from use by many countries after it was found to cause liver cancer in rats.

DIAZOLIDINYL UREA
A broad-spectrum antibacterial preservative used in cosmetics and personal-care products (with particularly good activity against Pseudomonas species). It is a formaldehyde-releasing preservative that, when mixed with nitrosating agents in the

product (see Appendix 1 for more), can form carcinogenic nitrosamines. It is also a sensitising agent that can provoke contact dermatitis.

DIBUTYLPHTHALATE
See *Phthalates*

DIETHANOLAMINE
DEA
A solvent, emulsifying agent, detergent, dispersing agent and humectant found in cosmetics and body-care products. Irritating to skin and mucous membranes. *DEA* is used in relatively few products but *DEA*-containing compounds including *Cocamide DEA, Cocamide MEA, DEA-cetyl phosphate, DEA oleth-3 phosphate, DEA lauryl sulphate, Lauramide DEA, Myristamide DEA, Oleamide DEA*, are very widely used.

While DEA by itself is not harmful it can react with other ingredients known as formaldehyde-formers in the product to form a potent carcinogen called *nitrosodiethanolamine (NDEA)*. NDEA is readily absorbed through the skin and has been linked with stomach, oesophageal, liver and bladder cancers. Related compounds such as *TEA lauryl sulphate* and *Triethanolamine*, can also mix synergistically with other ingredients to form *NDEA* in cosmetics (see Appendix 1 for more).

DIETHYL PHTHALATE
See *Phthalates*

DIETHYLHEXYL PHTHALATE
See *Phthalates*

DIMETHICONE
Film former, antifoaming agent and skin conditioner based on silicone, found in oiletries and cosmetics. film-formersmake the product more spreadable and can make skin feel smooth but they also trap other substances (including other ingredients in the product) beneath them. Because they do not allow the skin to breathe they may exacerbate skin irritation caused by sweat or by other substances. See also *Silicones*.

DIMETHICONE COPOLYOL
A more waterproof form of *Dimethicone* that sticks to skin and hair better. It is a polymer based on silicone, used as a conditioner in hair care products and as a skin protectant. It is not considered toxic, but with prolonged use it can make the skin look dull. See also *Silicones*.

DIMETHYL ETHER
Dimethyl oxide, Wood ether, *Methyl ether*
Found in hairsprays and other toiletries in pressurised containers. A relative of *propylene glycol*, is a solvent that it is easily absorbed through the skin. Once in the body it can bioaccumulate and is know to be a reproductive toxin.

DIMETHYLPHTHALATE
See *Phthalates*

DIMETHYLPOLYSILOXANE
See *Silicones*

DIOCTYL ADIPATE
Adipic acid
Plasticiser and solvent found in bath oils, eye shadow, foundations, cologne, blusher, nail-polish remover, perfumes, moisturizers and fake tanning preparations. Studies show it can migrate from the wrapping material into food. Applied topically it can be irritating to skin and eyes. With regular ingestion it is considered a possible human carcinogen, animal-based studies that show an increased incidence of liver tumours.

DIOXANE
Diethylene dioxide, Diethylene ether, Diethylene oxide
Found primarily as a contaminant in a variety of toiletry, cosmetic and household products, *dioxane* is a hazardous air pollutant and carcinogen. It is most often a contaminant in ethoxylated surfactants, detergents, foaming agents, emulsifiers and certain solvents. These ingredients are identifiable by the prefix, *PEG*, or words like *polyethylene, polyethylene glycol, polyoxyethylene*, or syllables such as '-eth-' or '-oxynol-'.

DIOXYBENZONE
A chemical used in sunscreen to block UVB. It is a derivative of *Benzophenone*.

DISODIUM EDTA
E386, Disodium ethylene-diamine-tetra-acetate
Preservative and antioxidant used in foods, cosmetics and household cleaners. In cosmetics and other formulations its purpose is to prevent the ingredients in a given formula from binding with trace elements (particularly minerals and metal impurities) and thereby changing the texture, odour and consistency of the product. If ingested or absorbed into the body can concentrate these impurities in the body. In the environment, they concentrate heavy metals and other contaminants in soil and the water supply. Applied topically it is irritating to eyes and skin and acts as a penetration enhancer.

DMDM HYDANTOIN
Diemethylol dimethyl hydantoin
A water-soluble preservative used in cosmetics. It can act as a formaldehyde-releasing agent. Should not be combined with *DEA* or *DEA*-containing compounds as this can cause the carcinogenic substance *NDELA* to form. See *Diethanolamine*.

ETHYL ALCOHOL
Ethanol
See *Alcohol*

ETHYL DIHYDROXYPROPYL PABA
See *PABAs*

ETHYL LINALOOL
See *Linalool*

ETHYLHEXYL P-METHOXYCINNAMATE
See *Cinnamates*

ETHYLHEXYL SALICYLATE
Octyl salicylate
See *Salicylates*

ETHYLPARABEN
See *Parabens*

EUGENOL
Synthetic fragrance in cosmetics. Also used as a fungicide and insecticide. A skin irritant and allergen in cosmetics. Poorly studied with regard to human safety but known to cause tumours in rats.

FLUORIDE
Sodium fluoride, Sodium monofluorophosphate
Added to toothpastes and to water to prevent dental caries. Fluoride falls somewhere between arsenic and lead in terms of its toxicity. When containers of fluoride arrive at the doors of toothpaste manufacturer they do so with a skull and crossbones on the on the front. Fluoride is a systemic poison and there is enough of this substance in a half a tube of family toothpaste to kill a small child.

Fluoride works best applied topically, but toothpaste rarely stays on the teeth long enough to be totally effective and its benefits are highly contested and continually overstsated. Ten years ago fluoride was touted as reducing the incidence of dental caries by 40–60 per cent; today the revised figure is 18–25 per cent. Levels of caries tend to be lowest in non-fluoridated areas and better diets and more conscientious brushing, are the likely major factor in our improved dental health.

While there is very little concrete evidence that fluoride genuinely protects teeth, there is plenty of evidence to show that regular exposure can cause harm. Studies have shown a clear relationship between oral cancers and fluoride intake in both animals and humans. Benign squamous papilloma, for instance, which appears as a white patch on the inside of the mouth and is the precursor of squamous cell carcinoma, can be triggered by fluoride exposure.

Fluoride can cause sensitivity/allergic type reactions and is now suspected in a host of illnesses including gastroesophageal reflux disease (GERD), bone problems, diabetes, thyroid malfunction and mental impairment. Fluoride exposure from toothpaste, supplements and water before the age of six is also an important risk factor for dental fluorisis, which mottles and discolours the teeth.

FORMALDEHYDE

Disinfectant, germacide, fungicide, defoamer and preservative. It is not used in foods, but can be used to disinfect containers, pipes and vessels in the food industry. It is widely used in personal-care products such including shampoo, nail polish and hardeners. Formaldehyde vapours are common indoor pollutants and are suspected human carcinogens that alter your sense of smell and can cause respiratory irritation. Anyone with asthma, lung infections or similar ailments can be severely affected by exposure to formaldehyde. It can also cause stuffy nose and itchy or watery eyes, nausea, headache and fatigue.

G-TERPINENE

Synthetic fragrance commonly found in cologne, perfume, soap, shaving cream, deodorant and air freshener. It can trigger asthma and is a central nervous system disrupter that can cause symptoms such as headache, mood swings, depression, incoordination and lethargy.

GERANIOL

Synthetic fragranc found in cosmetics, soaps, detergents, creams, lotions and air fresheners. This chemical is also used as a synthetic flavouring agent in beverages, ice cream and candies. It is also sometimes found in 'natural' pesticides to repel mosquitoes, flies, cockroaches, ants, gnats and ticks. Irritating to skin and eyes; a sensitiser and neurotoxin.

GLYCERIDES

Formed from a mixture of fatty acids and glycerol, glycerides have a variety of uses. In cosmetics they are often used as emulsifiers and emollients in soaps and detergents as well as moisturisers. Generally presumed to be safe.

GLYCERIN
Glycerol

A form of alcohol used as a solvent, humectant and lubricant in cosmetics. Glycerine can be processed from plants or animals. Prolonged contact can dry the skin (in common with other humectants such as *PEGs*) glycerine draws moisture from the closest most abundant source. If you live and/or work in a dry in environment the closest source of moisture will be your skin.

GLYCERYL PABA
See *PABA*

GLYCERYL STEARATE

An emulsifying wax made from hardened vegetable oil and glycerin with an addition of vegetable stearic acid. Generally considered safe, though it can provoke allergic reactions or contact dermatitis in some individuals.

GLYCOLIC ACID

See *Alpha hydroxy acids*

HEXYL LAURATE

Dodecanoic acid, Lauric acid
Synthetic flavouring and fragrance. Largely unevaluated for its effects on humans.

HEXYLCINNAMALDEHYDE

See *Cinnamates*

HEXYLENE GLYCOL

Used as a humectant, plasticiser, solvent and emulsifier in cosmetics. Can cause skin irritation in some individuals. Vapours can be irritating to the eyes and lungs. In animals, repeated ingestion or skin applications have been shown to affect the kidneys and liver.

HOMOSALATE

See *Salycilates*

HYALURONIC ACID

Hyaluronan
Used in skincare products as a moisturiser and humectant. *Hyaluronic acid* occurs naturally throughout the body and is an important component of connective tissue. The synthetic nature-identical version used in cosmetics provides little more than a temporary boost to ageing skin. It appears to be safe, although it has not been fully evaluated for safety in humans.

HYDRATED SILICA

Amorphous silica
Silica gel comprised of *Crystaline silica* in a watery matrix. Used in pharmaceutical and personal-care products as carriers for active ingredients, dispersants for colours and dyes and anticaking agents. Also uses as an abrasive and stain remover found in toothpastes and cleaning products. While it is the crystalline form of silica that is considered carcinogenic when inhaled, wet formulations contain these same particles. Used on teeth it can weaken tooth enamel and damage gums. In rare cases the silica can build up under the gum causing inflammation that mimics gingivitis. The safety of ingested silica has not been adequately proven and some observers have linked it with Crohn's disease, though this remains unsubstantiated (see also *Silica*).

HYDROFLUOROCARBONS
HCFCs

Propellants. Although they were introduced primarily as substitutes for ozone-depleting *chlorofluorocarbons* (CFCs), HFCs remain in the atmosphere for decades to centuries and are damaging greenhouse gases hastening the phenomenon of global climate change.

HYDROGEN PEROXIDE

Disinfectant, bleaching and oxidising agent found in toiletries (such as hair dyes) and household cleaners. Safe in very dilute mixtures. But at higher strengths can irritate the eyes, skin and mucous membranes; has been shown to be mutagenic in laboratory tests and carcinogenic in animals.

HYDROGENATED CASTOR OIL

Castor oil which has been thickened with the addition of hydrogen atom. It improves the feel of the cosmetic products such as body lotions, but can be a contact allergen.

HYDROXYCAPRILIC ACID

See *Alpha hydroxy acids*

HYDROXYCITRONELLOL

Synthetic floral fragrance. It is a contact allergen, skin, eye and lung irritant.

IMIDAZOLIDINYL UREA

A broad-spectrum antibacterial preservative with particularly good activity against Pseudomonas species. After parabens, it is the most commonly used cosmetic preservative. Found in cosmetics, baby shampoos, personal-care products and fragrances. It is a sensitising agent and a primary cause of contact dermatitis. It can release formaldehyde into the formulation and is most dangerous when used in combination with *ethanolamines* (ingredient names containing the acronyms *DEA*, *MEA* and *TEA*).

ISO E SUPER

Synthetic floral, woody fragrance. Similar in structure to synthetic musk compounds and may have similarly devastating, hormone-disrupting health effects.

ISOBUTANE

Propellant used in cosmetics, household and garden products and foods. Chronic exposure can produce a range of central nervous system symptoms such as headache, breathing difficulties, mood swings, nausea, vomiting, dizziness and symptoms mimicking drunkenness. Isobutane is a highly inflammable volatile organic chemical (VOC) popular with solvent abusers because they produce a quick 'high' – however it can also produce convulsions, coma and a quick death. VOCs also accumulate in human breast milk. While isobutane doesn't destroy the earth's ozone shield, it does contribute to the formation of ground-level ozone, or smog, which can cause serious breathing problems. See also *Butane* and *Propane*.

ISOBUTYLPARABEN
See *Parabens*

ISOEUGENOL
See *Eugenol*

ISOPROPANOL
See *Isopropyl alcohol*

ISOPROPYL ALCOHOL
Solvent found in glass cleaners and windshield-wiper solutions. Irritates eyes and mucous membranes and causes central nervous system depression. Prolonged contact can cause eczema and sensitisation. Animal studies show inhalation can damage the liver; ingestion results in drowsiness, unconsciousness and death.

ISOPROPYL PALMITATE
Palmitic acid, Hexadecanoic acid
Used in cosmetics as a thickening agent and emollient. Can be synthetic or derived from the palmitic acid in coconut oil. It is often used in moisturizes where it forms a thin layer and easily penetrates the skin. It can potentially clog pores.

ISOTRIDECYL SALICYLATE
See *Salicylates*

KATHON CG
A preservative compound widely used in cosmetics. It is a mixture of two synthetic chemicals *Methylchloroisothiazolinone* and *Methylisothiazolinone*. It is a contact allergen and sensitiser. *Methylisothiazolinone* has recently been identified as a neurotoxin that can damage nerve endings with repeated exposure.

LANOLIN
Derived from wool fat and used as an emollient and thickener in a wide range of cosmetics, hair products, ointments and lotions. Lanolin itself is non-toxic and unlikely to cause adverse effects, but impurities mixed in with it can cause allergic skin rashes.

LAURAMIDE DEA
See *Diethanolamine*

LAURETH COMPOUNDS
Ingredients such as *Laureth-7, Laureth 10* and *Laureth 23* are commonly used as emulsifiers in cosmetic products. These compounds are what are known as

'ethoxylated alcohols' and due to the way they are processed they can be contaminated with the carcinogen *1,4-dioxane*.

LAURIC ACID
Dodecanoic acid
The major fatty acid found in coconut oil or palm kernel oil, lauric acid is a common ingredient in many cosmetics, soaps and detergents. Generally regarded as safe.

LILIAL
A synthetic fragrance known to cause sentitisation when applied topically and immune suppression after inhalation.

LIMONENE
Synthetic citrus fragrance found in perfumes colognes, personal-care product and household cleaners and air fresheners and as a common pesticide in flea-control products. Can cause skin and eye irritation. May trigger asthma attacks and is a powerful sensitiser. Produces tumours, reproductive abnormalities and delayed growth in some animals.

LINALOOL
Synthetic herbal/woody fragrance found in perfumes colognes, personal-care product and household cleaners and air fresheners. It is also a common pesticide in flea control products. Can cause skin, eye and respiratory irritation. It has a narcotic effect in high doses and has been shown to cause central nervous system disorders in animals with symptoms of altered mood, poor muscular coordination and reduced spontaneous motor activity. Exposure can cause fatal respiratory disturbances. It attracts bees (thus poses a threat to people who are allergic to bee stings).

METHYL HEPTINE CARBONATE
Synthetic fragrance used in perfumes and air fresheners to impart a fresh, sweet, green, fruity scent. It is frequent cause of skin sensitisation and may trigger breathing difficulties.

METHYLCHLOROISOTHIAZOLINONE
Cosmetic preservative, usually combined with *Methylisothiazolinone* (this compound is known as *Kathon CG*). It is a strong allergen that binds quickly to the skin remaining there long after use. Laboratory studies suggest it is a potential mutagen and a suspected carcinogen due to its corrosive action on the skin.

METHYLISOTHIAZOLINONE
Cosmetic preservative usually combined with *Methylchloroisothiazolinone* (this combination is known as *Kathon CG*). It is a strong allergen that binds quickly to the skin remaining there long after use. Laboratory studies suggest this substance causes

the nerve damage. It is also a potential mutagen and a suspected carcinogen due to its corrosive action on the skin.

METHYLPARABEN
See *Parabens*

MICROBAN
See *Triclosan*

MINERAL OIL
See *Parafinnum liquidum*

MONOETHANOLAMINE
2-aminoethanol
Surfactant found in wash-off toiletries. Relative of *Diethanoamine*. Often denoted by the prefix or suffix *MEA* as in *Cocamide MEA*, *Linoleamide MEA* and *Stearamide MEA*. A skin and eye irritant. Inhaling *MEA* can irritate the lungs and trigger asthma attacks. It is also a gastrointestinal, liver and nervous system toxin.

MURIATIC ACID
See *Hydrochloric acid*

MYRISTAMINDE DEA
See *Diethanolamine*

N-BUTANE
See *Butane*

NITROPHENYLENEDIAMINE
See *Phenylenediamines*

OCTOCRYLENE
See *Cinnamates*

OCTYL METHOXYCINNAMATE
See *Cinnamates*

OCTYL SALICYLATE
See *Salicylates*

OLEAMIDE DEA
See *Diethanolamine*

OLETH

Cosmetic emulsifiers and surfactants denoted by names such as *Oleth-5* and *Oleth-2*. They can produce allergic skin reactions and because they are in the same family as *PEG* compounds they may contain impurities linked to breast cancer (e.g. *1,4-dioxane, ethylene oxide*). Toxic to aquatic organisms.

ORTHO-AMINOPHENOL

Found in permanent and semi-permanent hair dyes it imparts a light brown colour to hair. A derivative of *p-phenylenediamine* (see *Phenylendiamines*).

ORTHO-PHENYLENEDIAMINE

See *Phenylenediamines*

OXYBENZONE

See *Benzophenones*

PABA

Para-aminobenzoic acid

PABA and its related compounds such as *ethyl dihydroxypropyl PABA, padimate-O (ocyl dimethyl PABA), padimate A* and *glyceryl PABA* are used as sunscreening agents. Applied topically they can cause skin irritation and sensitization as well as producing light sensitivity (with blistering and peeling skin) in some individuals. *PABAs* are formaldehyde-forming chemicals that can form carcinogenic nitrosamines when combined with amines such as *DEA, TEA* and *MEA* in the mixture. *PABAs* can cause skin irritation. *PABA's* are relatives of the cosmetic preservatives parabens (see separate listing) and in addition to being irritating to the skin are also thought to be oestrogenic.

PADIMATE-A

Amyl Dimethylaminobenzoate
See *PABA*

PADIMATE-O

Octyl dimethyl PABA
See *PABA*

PALMITIC ACID

Emollient, moisturiser and emulsifier found in a wide range of cosmetics. Can cause contact dermatitis in some individuals.

PARA-AMINOBENZOIC ACID

See *PABA*

PARA-AMINOPHENOL

Reddish-brown colour found in hair dyes. Must be mixed with an oxidising agent (e.g. hydrogen peroxide, *resorcinol*) to produce the required colour. Can trigger moderate to severe skin reactions in some individuals. Once in the body it can cause kidney damage.

PARABENS

Butylparaben, ethylparaben, isobutylparaben, methylparaben, propylparaben
The most widely used group of preservatives found in cosmetics. It is estimated that more than 90 per cent of all cosmetic products contain some form of parabens.

Applied topically they can cause skin irritation, contact dermatitis and contact allergies Animal and laboratory studies have long shown that parabens have a weak oestrogenic activity. *Butylparaben* and *isobutylparaben* have the strongest hormonal effect followed by *propylparaben*, *ethylparaben* and *methylparaben*. Whether this poses any health risk for humans is still unclear. In animal studies, ingested parabens can induce cell proliferation (often a precursor of ·cancer) in the forestomach and birth defects in mice and rats. Recently, when scientists conducted an analysis of breast cancer tissue they found accumulated parabens in every sample examined. The researchers suggested that parabens in deodorants and antiperspirants could be the cause.

Our bodies are exposed to oestrogens from many sources and it is possible that regularly ingesting or absorbing weak oestrogens from a number of different sources may add up to a strong oestrogenic effect in the body. Too much oestrogen in the body is a trigger for oestrogen-dependent cancers of the breast, ovary, uterus and testicles and may even have effects on foetal development. Although parabens are used in small amounts in individual products, they are widely used in all toiletries and cosmetics – usually in products that are left on for long periods of time. It is likely that we absorb parabens from each of the products we use. Thus parabens need to be viewed in the light of the larger problem of exposure to environmental oestrogens.

PARAFFINUM LIQUIDUM

Mineral oil, Baby oil
A transparent, odourless and colourless oil derived from petroleum. In cosmetics it is an emollient and film former. Ingested it can inhibit the absorption of essential fats and have a mild laxative effect. A human carcinogen and reproductive toxin if inhaled. In cosmetics it is a used as an emollient to produce a temporary moisturising effect. However, prolonged use destroys the natural oily barrier of the skin leading to more persistent dryness. By destroying the protective oily barrier of the skin, mineral oil also acts like a penetration enhancer allowing other chemicals to be more easily absorbed into the skin and bloodstream. If inhaled it can cause fatal pneumonia. In the US products containing mineral oil are obliged to carry a warning and also to have child-proof caps.

Manufacturers have slowly been replacing the mineral oil in their products with other synthetics such as Silicones.

PARA-PHENYLENEDIAMINE

p-Phenylenediamine

Black colour found in hair dyes. Must be mixed with an oxidising agent (e.g. hydrogen peroxide, *resorcinol*) to produce the required colour. Can trigger moderate to severe skin reactions in some individuals. Once in the body it can cause kidney damage. See also *Phenylenediamines*.

PARA-TOLUENEDIAMINE

p-Toluenediamine

Brown colour found in hair dyes. Must be mixed with an oxidising agent (e.g. hydrogen peroxide, resorcinol) to produce the required colour. Can trigger moderate to severe skin reactions in some individuals. Once in the body it can cause liver damage. Belongs to a family of dyes and intermediaries known as *Diaminotoulenes*.

PARETH

A surfactant that belongs to the same family as *Polyethylene glycol*.

PARFUM

Perfume, fragrance

'Parfum' is the collective name given to hundreds of different chemicals used to produce a fragrance in cosmetics and toiletries. Perfumes contain every kind of poison known to man, which is why many perfume ingredients double up as pesticides. Most, for instance, are solvents and as such as are damaging to the brain and nervous system (neurotoxic). Many are persistent (i.e. they don't break down in the environment and they accumulate in human tissue and breastmilk) and can cause birth defects. Artificial musks, a common ingredient in fragranced toiletries, are hormone disrupting and cancer causing. Immediate reactions to parfum include headache, mood swings, depression, forgetfulness and irritation. It is also a major trigger of attacks in asthmatics. Of the 20 most common perfume ingredients, four – *acetone, ethanol, ethyl acetate, methylene chloride* – are classified as hazardous waste by the EPA. Spray formulations mean you – and those around you – inhale more of these toxic chemicals.

PEG

Polyethylene glycol

Polyethylene glycol (*PEG*) compounds are derived from natural gas and have numerous functions in toiletries including: moisturisers, emulsifiers, emollients, antioxidants, plasticizers, solvents and softeners. Adding *PEG* to a product will also prevent moisture loss during storage.

On the ingredients label, *PEG*s are usually listed followed by a number (e.g. *PEG-4* or *PEG-350*) that refers to its molecular weight. These number represent the liquidity of the compound; the higher the number, the more solid it is. *PEG* compounds can be contaminated with the carcinogen *1,4-dioxane*. They can also form carcinogens when mixed with *DEA* and *TEA* compounds (see Appendix 1).

PETROLATUM
Petroleum jelly, Vaseline

This chemical lubricant is derived from petroleum. Used to make skin creams feel smoother. Can provoke allergic skin reactions and over time will destroy the natural oily barrier on the skin leaving it more prone to drying, flaking and cracking.

PHENOXYETHANOL
Cosmetic preservative that can cause skin irritation, contact dermatitis and contact allergies.

PHENOXYISOPROPANOL
Preservative and solvent found in acne treatments, shampoos and facial cleansers. A strong irritant that can only be used in wash-off products. Skin reactions are likely.

PHENYLENEDIAMINES
A family of dyes commonly found in permanent and semi-permanent hair colours. They can damage skin, cause allergic reactions (sometimes fatal) and are irritating to the eyes. *Phenylenediamines* are also carcinogenic, can cause immune-system dysregulation as well as kidney and liver damage. They are toxic to wildlife and soil. The type of *phenylenediamine* used depends on the end colour, thus:

- para-phenylenediamine (black)
- para-toluenediamine (brown)
- ortho-phenylenediamine (brown)
- para-aminophenol (reddish brown)
- ortho-aminophenol (light brown)

PHENYL-P-PHENYLENEDIAMINE
See *Phenylenediamines*

PHTHALATES
Phthalates are a class of widely used industrial compounds that have become ubiquitous, not just in the products in which they are intentionally used, but also as contaminants in almost everything. They can be used as softeners in plastics, oily substances in perfumes and additives to hairsprays, lubricants and wood finishers. Phthalates are oestrogen mimics that can easily leech out of the products in our homes. Animal studies show that exposure to very low levels of the phthalates *dibutyl phthalate* (*DBP*) and *diethylhexyl phthalate* (*DEHP*) in the womb caused demasculinization of male foetuses and increased the rate of reproductive disorders such as *hypospadias* (where the urethra opens on the underside of the penis). *Phthalate* exposure is also linked to reduction in sperm quality.

POLYCYCLIC AROMATIC HYDROCARBONS
Polycyclic aromatic hydrocarbons (PAHs) are a group of over 100 different chemicals

created by incineration of plastic waste such as polyvinyl chloride (PVC), high-density polyethylene (HDPE) and polypropylene as well as other industrial waste. They are found in asphalt, creosote, coal-tar pitch, roofing tar, coal and crude oil. A few are used in medicines, plastics, dyes and pesticides.

Animal studies have also shown that PAHs can have harmful effects on the skin, body fluids and immune system after both short- and long-term exposure. Mice exposed to high levels of PAHs during pregnancy had difficulty reproducing, and so did their offspring. These offspring also had higher rates of birth defects and lower body weights. In laboratory animals, PAHs ingested and inhaled and applied to the skin produced a variety of cancers.

POLYETHYLENE GLYCOL
See *PEGs*

POLYOXYETHYLENE ALKYL ETHERS
Family of detergents, surfactants and wetting agents found in household cleaning products and cosmetics. *Lauryl alcohol* and *cetyl alcohol* as well as *sorbitan* are *polyoxyethylene* compounds found n cosmetics and in toiletries as an emulsifying agent. In household cleaning products, compounds like *nonyl phenol* are used because of their strong degreasing effects. Some *polyoxyethylene* compounds are also used as fabric softeners and antistatic agents. They are mostly non-irritating but can be contaminated with the *carcinogen 1,4-dioxane*.

POLYSORBATES
Emulsifiers and surfactans used in foods and cosmetics. Belong to a large group of chemicals known as *Polyoxyethylene alkyl ethers*. Can be contaminated with the carcinogen *1,4-dioxane*.

POLYTETREFLUOROETHYLENE
PTFE, Teflon
See *Teflon*

POLYVINYLPYRROLIDONE
Clarifying additive in wine, beer and vinegar, also used in the production of dietary supplements. *PVP* compounds can also be found in hair styling products, especially hairsprays. Inhalation of *PVP* damages the lungs; animal studies suggest it is associated with damage to the kidneys and liver as well as an increased risk of cancer when ingested.

POTASSIUM HYDROXIDE
Caustic potash, Lye
Harsh alkalai used as an intermediate in soap production and as a neutraliser in food production. Also found in nail cuticle softeners and depilatories. It is corrosive to the eyes, mucous membranes and skin and can cause dermatitis and burns even in dilute solutions.

PPG-3 METHYL ETHER
See *Propylene glycol*

PPG-14 BUTYL ETHER
See *Propylene glycol*
Used primarily in cosmetics as a preservative, solvent *PPG-14 butyl ether* is a relative of *propylene glycol* and in addition to being a skin irritant and neurotoxin it is potentially toxic to the kidney and liver. In the US it is a pesticide component used in sprays to protect animals from flies, gnats and mosquitoes. It is poisonous in high concentrations and can enhance the skin penetration of other more toxic chemicals.

PROPANE
Petroleum derived propellant for aerosol sprays, especially after the ban of *Chlorofluorocarbons* (*CFCs*). Skin contact may result in frostbite and burns. A central nervous system toxicant that can produce symptoms rapid breathing, incoordination, rapid fatigue, excessive salivation, disorientation, headache, nausea and vomiting.

PROPYLENE GLYCOL
PPG, 1,2-Propanediol
Solvent, humectant and wetting agent found in foods, cosmetics and household products. Irritating to eyes, skin and respiratory tract. Applied topically it acts as a penetration enhancer, altering skin structure, allowing other more toxic chemicals to penetrate more deeply into the skin and eventually the bloodstream.

PVP
See *Polyvinylpyrollidone*

QUATERNARY AMMONIUM COMPOUNDS
A large family of strong disinfectants and surfactants found in household cleaners but also in some medications such as ophthalmic preparations and in cosmetics. Highly toxic and implicated in the rise of drug resistant bacteria in homes and hospitals. In eye drops they can damage eyes on contact. Examples of quaternary ammonium compounds include *Benzalkonium chloride*, *Alkyl triethanol ammonium chloride*, *Benzethonium chloride* and *Cetrimide* (*cetyltrimethylammonium bromide*).
In cosmetics they are used as preservatives, examples of which include: *quaternium-15*, *quaternium 18* and *quaternium-80*. Applied to the skin they can be irritating and because they are formaldehyde-forming compounds they can produce carcinogenic nitrosamines when mixed with *DEA* and *TEA* (See Appendix 1).

RED PETROLATUM
A reddish-brown, grease-like petroleum jelly. Its natural pigments are effective in blocking the sun's ultraviolet rays, During WWII, red petrolatum was extensively used by the military. Largely fallen out of fashion but still used as a sunblock in some products

RESORCINOL

1,3-benzenediol, m-dihydroxybenzene, resorcin

Oxidizing agent commonly found in permanent and semi-permanent hair dyes. It is also used as an anti-dandruff agent in shampoo, sunscreen products as well as in pesticide formulations. Resorcinol fights fungal and bacterial organisms and promotes softening, dissolution and peeling of the skin and is sometimes used to treat acne eczema, psoriasis, corns, calluses, warts and other skin conditions. Irritating to eyes and skin; can cause contact allergies. Resorcinol may be absorbed into the body through the skin and into the bloodstream where it acts like a hormone-disruptor linked to reproductive effects thyroid damage, central nervous system effects, including dizziness, nausea, altered heartbeat and restlessness.

SALICYLATES

Vast range of chemicals that can be used as flavourings and aromas in foods (e.g. *amyl, phenyl, menthyl* and *glyceryl salicylate*) and as perfume ingredients in fragranced cosmetics and household products (e.g. *benzyl salicylate, CIS-3-hexenyl salicylate*). One of their most wide spread uses is cosmetics is as sunscreening agents, (e.g. *homosalate, ethylhexyl salicylate, octyl salicylate, isotridecyl salicylate* and *trolamine salicylate*). People who are sensitive to aspirin may develop allergic-type reactions from ingesting *salicylates* or applying them to the skin. In addition *salicylates* are penetration enhancers that allow other chemicals in the product to get deeper into the bloodstream; research also shows that some *salicylates* used in suncreams are oestrogenic.

SALICYLIC ACID

Used as a preservative in food products and cosmetics. Also a common dandruff treatment in shampoos. In anti-ageing creams salicylic acid is a *Beta hydroxy acid*, used as a chemical peel to dissolve and removing the outer layer of skin. Because of its exfoliating action, salicylic acid can increase photosensitivity of the skin and cause contact dermatitis. See also *Salicylates*.

SELENIUM SULPHIDE

Anti-dandruff agent that is irritating to the skin and eyes. Avoid contact with broken skin.

SILICA

A natural mineral (*silicon dioxide*) used as an anticaking agent in salts and salt substitutes and other dry food items. In cosmetics it is used as an abrasive, absorbent and viscosity adjuster. Inhaling silica dust is a risk factor in developing lung cancer (see *Crystlaine silica, Hydrated silica*).

SILICATES

A family of naturally-occurring, quartz-containing minerals (e.g. silica). In dry form they are used in powder bases for cosmetics such as face powder, eye shadow or blusher. Magnesium silicate, or *talc* is a good example of a silicate used for this purpose. Other types of powdered silicates are used as abrasives in toothpastes and household cleaners. Inhaling silica dust is a risk factor in developing lung cancer.

SILICONES

Any group of semisynthetic fluid oils, rubbers and resins derived from silica (e.g. *Dimethicone, Simethicone*). Widely used in cosmetics as film formers, skin conditioning agents and water repellents. Generally considered safe, though poorly studied with regard to toxicity in humans.

SIMETHICONE

Synthetic silicone-based moisturiser and filmformer used in cosmetics. Film-formers trap other substances (including other ingredients in the product) beneath them. Because they do not allow the skin to breathe they may exacerbate skin irritation caused by sweat or by other substances.

SODIUM BICARBONATE

Baking soda

Often usedin toothpastes as a whitening/bleaching agent. Can be a harsh abrasive if used in concentrated form. Generally regarded as safe.

SODIUM COCOATE

Detergent derived from coconut oil. Generally considered mild and safe.

SODIUM COCOYL ISETHIONATE

A detergent/surfactant made from entirely synthetic sources that can be irritating to the skin.

SODIUM CHLORIDE

Salt

Simple table salt, a water softener added to help the product rinse better in hard water. Used in cosmetics and household cleaners ad a viscosity adjuster (thickener).

SODIUM FLUORIDE

See *Fluoride*

SODIUM LAURETH SULPHATE

SLES

A detergent and foaming agent found bath foams, bubble baths and shampoos. Can be irritating to eyes and skin. Laureth compounds can be contaminated with the carcinogen *1,4-dioxane*.

SODIUM LAURYL SULPHATE
SLS

A detergent and foaming agent found bath foams, bubble baths, shampoos and toothpastes. *SLS* is not carcinogenic but it can be damaging. It is so harsh that it is used in medical research to induce a kind of benchmark skin irritation against which all other potential skin irritants can be measured. If used in toothpastes, it is damaging to the delectate mucousal lining of the mouth, if it gets into the eyes during shampooing it can damage the cornea. Because it strips the protective oily layer from the skin it can also act as a penetration enhancer, making it easier for other toxic chemicals to be absorbed into the body.

As new detergents have been invented, the popularity of *SLS* among manufacturers has waned, but it is still in many products and often its presence is a good indicator of other undesirable ingredients, including formaldehyde-containing preservatives (e.g., *imidazolidinyl urea*) and nitrosamine-forming agents (e.g. *cocamide DEA*, *triethanolamine*) as well as a long list of skin and hair conditioners necessary to repair some of the initial damage it causes.

SODIUM LAUROAMPHOACETATE
Detergent/surfactant found in body washes and shampoos. Comparatively mild, so often found in sensitive or no-tears baby shampoos.

SODIUM MONOFLUOROPHOSPHATE
See *Fluoride*

SODIUM PALM KERNELATE
A detergent synthesised from the oil of palm kernels, usually found in soap and bath bars. Generally non-toxic.

SODIUM PALMATE
A detergent synthesised from the oil of palm kernels, usually found in soap and bath bars. Generally non-toxic.

SODIUM STEARATE
Found in shampoos and facial washes. It is a fatty acid added in its capacity as a skin softener to replace the oils stripped away from the skin by the mix of detergents.

SODIUM TALLOWATE
A detergent synthesised from animal fats found in facial and bath soaps. Generally non-toxic.

SORBITAN LAURATE
Emulsifier and surfactant used in cosmetics. Generally mild but it can cause skin irritation in some.

SORBITAN OLEATE

Used in cosmetics as an emulsifier and surfactant synthesised from olive oil. Generally mild but it can cause skin irritation in some.

SORBITAN STEARATE

A modified fatty acid derived from beef tallow. It is used as an emulsifier, stabiliser and surfactant in cosmetics. Generally mild but it can cause blackheads in some individuals.

SOYTRIMONIUM CHLORIDE

A Quaternary ammonium compound used as a surfactant and detergent in foaming bath products and shampoos. Toxic by all routes of exposure. Skin and airway irritation are common. Depending on the concentration, quaternary compounds may also produce nausea, vomiting, abdominal pain, anxiety, restlessness, coma, convulsions and respiratory muscle paralysis.

STEARAMIDE MEA

See *Monoethanolamine*

STEARAMIDOPROPYL DIMETHYLAMINE

Part of a larger group of glycol ethers (the same family as Propylene glycol and Polyethylene glycol compounds). *Glycol ethers* are solvents and wetting agents that are quickly absorbed into the skin. In the body they are reproductive toxins.

STEARETH

Waxy compounds (e.g. *Steareth-2*, *Steareth-21*) used as emulsifiers. They are part of a larger group of ethoxylated alcohols that are toxic and potentially carcinogenic in their own right and may be contaminated with the carcinogen *1,4-dioxane*.

STEARIC ACID

Lubricant and emulsifier derived from both animal and vegetable sources, added to soften. Found in shampoos and facial washes, it is a fatty acid added as skin softeners to replace the oils stripped away from the skin by the mix of detergents. Can be irritating to the skin, eyes and respiratory tract.

STEARYL ALCOHOL

Emollient, moisturiser and stabiliser derived from animal fats. Used as a lubricating agent to help the product go on more smoothly. It is thought to be non-toxic but can cause mild skin irritation and even contact dermatitis in sensitive individuals.

STRONTIUM CHLORIDE

Added to some toothpastes to reduce periodontal disease. Also found in some treatment shampoos and facial washes. Considered toxic and can be irritating to skin and mucous membranes.

SULISOBENZONE
Sunscreening agent. See *Benzophenones*

TALC
Magnesium silicate
Talc is made up of finely ground particles of stone. It is used widely in powdered cosmetics as well as an absorbent on its own. As it originates in the ground and is a mined product, it can be contaminated with other substances. Asbestos is a good example and recent reports about the talc used in crayon manufacture being contaminated with this poisonous substance have cause alarm to every parent whose child has ever sucked a crayon.

Regular use is also associated with respiratory problems in adults and children. Because it is comprised of finely ground stone it can lodge in the lungs permanently. In women using it in the genital area, it has been linked to ovarian cancer; it is now estimated that women who frequently use talc have three times the risk of developing ovarian cancer compared to non-users.

TEA LAURYL SULPHATE
See *Triethanolamine*

TEA SODIUM LAURYL SULPHATE
See *Triethanolamine*

TEFLON
Polytetrafluoroethylene, PTFE
Non-stick coating on cookware and the packaging for fast- and microwaveable food such as French fries, popcorn and pizza, as well as confectionary wrappers and other products, waterproof coating on fabrics (where it is known as Stainmaster, Gore-Tex and Scotchguard) and film former used in cosmetics. According to the US Environmental Protection Agency one of the breakdown products of Teflon, known as *PFOA* (*Perfluorooctanoic acid*) is an expected human carcinogen. *PFOA* can be released when Teflon is heated and can cause severe respiratory distress (and is deadly to pet birds). It is a persistent chemical pollutant found in almost every animal on the planet including humans. As evidence of *PFOA*'s toxicity continues to accumulate, some observers believe that their effect on humans may yet make DDT look almost safe by comparison.

TETRASODIUM EDTA
Tetrasodium ethylenediamine tetra acetic acid
Cosmetic preservative used in soaps and other toiletries. It helps to isolate impurities such as metals which cause the mixture to degrade. Can cause skin, mucous membrane and eye irritation, as well as contact dermatitis and contact allergies. Also acts as a penetration enhancer. Environmentally persistent, it binds with heavy metals in lakes and streams which aids its re-entry into the food chain.

THIMEROSAL

Mercury-containing preservative found in certain cosmetics such as mascara as well as in ophthalmic preparations. Highly toxic, damaging to the eyes; may add to the body's burden of the neurotoxin mercury.

TITANIUM DIOXIDE

Titanium dioxide is extracted from the naturally occurring mineral Ilmenite. Also used as a colouring, opacifier and as a sunscreening agent in cosmetics. Thought not to be easily absorbed and generally considered safe used in topical formulations, ingestion can produce detectable amounts in the blood, brain and glands with the highest concentrations being in the lymph nodes and lungs. Banned in Germany.

TOLUENE

Toluol, Methylbenzene

Toluene and its chemical cousin *Xylene* are aromatic hydrocarbons used primarily as solvents. Commonly found in dry cleaning solutions and perfume. *Toluene* easily enters the body through inhalation and ingestion, but is poorly absorbed via the skin. Irritating to the skin and respiratory tract. It can cause damage to several organs including eyes, liver, kidneys and the central nervous system (where it acts like a narcotic). Symptoms of chronic exposure include fatigue, weakness, confusion, headache, watery eyes, muscular fatigue, insomnia, dermatitis and photosensitivity.

TRICLOSAN

2,4,4'-trichloro-2'-hydroxy diphenyl ether

An antibacterial agent found in household cleaners, toothpastes, mouthwashes, face washes and bath products. Applied to the skin it can cause allergic reactions and ulceration. In the mouth it kills both 'good' and 'bad' bacteria so makes users more vulnerable to infection. It can also cause premature cell death in the gingival tissues resulting in gum damage. Is easily absorbed into the body via the mouth and has been associated with liver damage and eye irritation. It is a *chlorophenol*, a class of chemicals that can cause cancer in animals. Commonly used as a pesticide, it is easily absorbed into the body via the mouth and has been associated with liver damage in animals. Widespread use of *Triclosan* in commercial products is also implicated in increasing rates of bacterial resistance.

TRIETHANOLAMINE

TEA

Surfactant, emulsifier, dispersant and pH adjuster commonly used in shampoos and foaming bath products. Can be irritating to the skin and eyes. More worryingly, it may, during storage on the skin or in the body after absorption, mix with formaldehyde forming chemicals in the product to form carcinogenic compounds called nitrosamines (see Appendix 1). *TEA* is also a suspected endocrine disrupter. Animal studies have demonstrated liver and kidney damage from chronic exposure.

TRIETHANOLAMINE LAURYL SULPHATE

See *Triethanolamin*

TRISODIUM EDTA

See *Tetrasodium EDTA*

UREA

Carbamide

Naturally found in urine and other body fluids, today it is synthesised from ammonia and carbon dioxide. Worldwide the most common use for urea is as a fertiliser. In skincare products it is used to soften, moisturise and smooth hardened skin. Generally regarded as safe although regular topical applications can cause thinning of the skin and may impair skin function.

VA/VINYL BUTYL BENZOATE/CROTONATES COPOLYMER

A petroleum-based vinyl acetate that forms a thin plastic-like film on the hair that aids styling. It can cause mild skin irritation.

VINYL ACETATE/ACRYLIC COPOLYMER

A petroleum-based vinyl acetate that forms a thin plastic-like film on the hair that aids styling. It can cause mild skin irritation.

XYLENE

Xylol, Dimethylbenzene

A chemical cousin of *Toluene* and an aromatic hydrocarbons used primarily as a solvent. Commonly found in dry cleaning solutions and perfume. *Xylene* easily enters the body through inhalation and ingestion, but is poorly absorbed via the skin. Irritating to the skin and respiratory tract. It can cause damage to several organs including eyes, liver, kidneys and the central nervous system (where it acts like a narcotic). Symptoms of chronic exposure include fatigue, weakness, confusion, headache, watery eyes, muscular fatigue, insomnia, dermatitis and photosensitivity.

ZINC OXIDE

Popular mineral-based sunblock. Generally considered safe and effective though in some individuals it can cause skin irritation.

ZINC STEARATE

Found in shampoos and facial washes it is a fatty acid added as skin softeners to replace the oils stripped away from the skin by the mix of detergents.

Resources

Natural and organic alternatives exist for almost every kind of conventional personal-care product you wish to use. In the UK currently spend around £800 million a year on natural cosmetics and toiletries. This figure represents around 16 per cent of the total market, and it is one that is growing all the time.

A recent survey in the US found that around 90 per cent of women want to use natural and organic body-care products, but fewer than half of these women could actually define what natural and organic meant.

That's not surprising given the way that some companies misrepresent these concepts to their customers. When it comes to toiletries, there is no clear, legal, definition for the words natural and organic. For instance, a product need only contain 1 per cent natural ingredients to be called 'natural'. A label can claim organic ingredients and yet still contain a range of synthetic industrial chemicals that are not good for your skin and have been linked with longer-term health problems. In this situation, it's easy to see how women could become mistrustful of any product that makes such claims.

If you are new to buying natural alternatives this list will give you some great ideas for where to start – from simple basics like soap to luxuries like natural perfumes. Some of these are brands that you can find in small specialist shops, health stores and increasingly supermarkets and department stores. Others are readily available online, making shopping for well-made products effortless.

Natural Brands

Including face, bath and body care, cosmetics, perfumes, dental care, deodorants, men's products, children's and baby products, and sun protection.(★ Indicates a luxury, more expensive brand.)

Akamuti
Face, body and hair care, soap, oils and essential oils, body balms and butters. Includes a babies' range.
www.akamuti.co.uk

Alqvimia★
Face and body care, bath and shower products, oils and perfume.
Available in the UK through www.thenaturalstore.co.uk and www.naturalskincarespa.co.uk

Aubrey Organics
Face, body and hair care, bath and shower, cosmetics, deodorants, sun protection. Includes a men's and babies' range.
www.aubreyorganicsuk.co.uk
In the US www.aubreyorganics.com

Avalon Organics
Face, body and hair care, bath and shower products and deodorant.
Available in the UK through www.auravita.com
In the US www.avalonorganics.com

Aveda
Hair care, face and body care, Men and 'Pure-fume'.
www.aveda.co.uk
In the US www.aveda.com

Bamford★
Face, body and hair care, bath oils, massage oils and a baby range
www.daylesfordorganic.com

Bentley Organic
Soaps, bodywash and haircare
www.bentleyorganic.com

Burt's Bees
Face and body care, cosmetics, lip care, soaps, and natural remedies, a baby range, natural insect repellent.
www.myburtsbees.co.uk

Barefoot Botanicals
Face and body care plus an 'SOS' range created for people with eczema or psoriasis.
www.barefoot-botanicals.com

Care★
Facecare from Stella McCartney
www.stellamccartneycare.com

Cornwall Soap Box
Face, body and hair care and hand-made soap
www.cornwallsoapbox.co.uk

Dr Bronner
Hemp-formulated multipurpose soaps, organic bars, lip balm and body-care products.
Available from many health and online stores in the UK.
See also www.21stcentury health.co.uk
In the US www.drbronner.com

Dr Hauschka
Face, bath, body and hair care, make up,
sun protection, deodorants, toothpaste
and mouthwash.
www.drhauschka.co.uk

Duchy Originals
Hair and body care, bath soak and
soaps.
www.duchyoriginals.com

Earthbound Organics
Face and body care, massage oils,
medicinal balms, creams and herbal
tinctures. Includes a babies' and
men's range.
www.earthbound.co.uk

Essential Care
Face, body and hair care, massage oils,
essential oils and 'Mum and Baby'
range.
www.essential-care.co.uk

Faith in Nature
Face, body and hair care and soaps.
www.faithinnature.com

Green People
Face, body and hair care, bath and
shower gel, cosmetics, soap, sun
protection and dental care. Includes a
men's, babies' and children's range.
www.greenpeople.co.uk

Ila★
Face oils, creams and masks, bath salts,
body scrubs, balms and oils.
www.ila-spa.com

Jo Wood Organics★
Bath oil, body lotion, body dew
and soap.
www.jowoodorganics.com

John Masters Organics★
Hair, Face and body care and soap.
www.johnmasters.co.uk
In the US www.johnmasters.com

Lavera
Face, body and hair care, 'bath spa'
range, cosmetics, sun protection,
products for men, babies and children,
wooden brushes and combs.
www.lavera.co.uk

My Being Well
Face, body and hair care, bath and
shower, men and mother and baby.
www.mybeingwell.com

Neal's Yard
Homeopathic remedies, herbal
supplements, oils, essential oils, natural
face, body and hair care, bath and
shower gels, soaps, deodorants, sun
protection, natural insect repellent.
www.nealsyardremedies.com

Nude★
Face and body care.
www.nudefacecare.com

Korres
Face, body and hair care, bath and
shower products, make up, men's range,
'young skin' range and suncare.
www.korres.com

Primavera
Face, body and hair care, bath and
shower products, massage and body oil,
treatment blends, eau de toilette,
men's range.
www.primavera.co.uk

Pure Nuff Stuff
Face, body and haircare, cosmetics, soaps, men's and baby range, deodorants and sun protection.
www.purenuffstuff.co.uk

Organic Blue
Body and hair care, bath oils, massage oils and men's range.
www.organicblue.com

REN★
Face, body and hair care, bath and shower and fragrance.
www.renfacecare.com

So Organic
Face, body and hair care, bath and shower, deodorants, dental care, men's range, babies' range, sun protection, sanitary products.
www.soorganic.com

Spiezia★
Face, body and haircare, bath, healing ointments, mother and baby, men's range.
www.spieziaorganics.com

The Organic Apoteke★
Face and body care, spa treatments and perfume.
www.organicapoteke.com

The Organic Pharmacy★
Face, body and haircare, make-up, sun protection, oils, homeopathic remedies, herbal tinctures, supplements, men's products, mother and baby care, detox at home kits.
www.theorganicpharmacy.com

Simply Soaps
Soaps, face, body and hair care, bath products, massage oils and natural insect repellent.
www.simplysoaps.com/uk

Suki★
Face, body and hair care and cosmetics
www.sukipureskincare.co.uk
In the US www.sukisnaturals.com

Trevarno
Face and body care, bath products, soothing ointments, soaps, sun care. Includes men's and babies' range.
www.trevarnoskincare.co.uk

Verde
Face and body care, bath products, special treatment creams and gels, oils, make up, men's range, mother and child.
www.verde.co.uk

Weleda
Face, body and hair care, medicines, dental care, sun protection, baby care.
www.weleda.co.uk

Wild Wood Groves
Argan-oil based face, body and hair care, includes a men's and babies' range.
www.wildwoodgroves.com

Willow
Face, body and hair care, bath and shower, fragrances, men's range.
www.willowbeautyproducts.co.uk

Make-up

Burt's Bees
www.myburtsbees.co.uk

Dr Hauschka
www.drhauschka.co.uk

Lavera
www.lavera.co.uk

Lily Lolo
www.lilylolo.co.uk

Purity Cosmetics
www.puritycosmetics.co.uk

Suki★
Face, body and hair care and cosmetics
www.sukipureskincare.co.uk
In the US www.sukisnaturals.com

Verde
www.verde.co.uk

Yaoh
Hemp-based face, body and hair care,
bath and shower, massage oil and sun
protection.
www.yaoh.co.uk

Products for men

Aubrey Organics
www.aubreyorganicsuk.co.uk
In the US www.aubreyorganics.com

Aveda
www.aveda.co.uk; or in the US
www.aveda.com

Green People
www.greenpeople.co.uk

Male Organics
www.male-organics.com

Verde
www.verde.co.uk

Deodorant

Green People
www.greenpeople.co.uk

PikRok Ltd
www.pitrok.co.uk

Tom's of Maine
www.tomsofmaine.com

Soap

Caurnie Soaperie
www.caurnie.com

Ecosoapia
www.ecosoapia.com

Toothpaste and mouthwash

Kingfisher Toothpaste
www.kingfishertoothpaste.com

Aloe Dent
www.optimah.com

Sarakan
www.sarakan.co.uk

Tom's of Maine
www.tomsofmaine.com

Perfumes

Alqvimia★
Available from
www.thenaturalstore.co.uk;
www.naturalskincarespa.co.uk

Aromasciences
www.aromasciences.com

Dolma
www.dolma-perfumes.co.uk

Farfalla
www.farfalla-essentials.co.uk; also
available from
www.thenaturalstore.co.uk

Florascent★
Available from
www.thenaturalstore.co.uk

Headonism
www.headonism.biz/headonism.html

Jo Wood★
www.jowoodorganics.com

Primavera
www.primavera.co.uk

Rich Hippie Perfumes★
Available in the UK from
www.thenaturalstore.co.uk
In the US www.rich-hippie.com

Wickle
Available from
www.thenaturalstore.co.uk

Hair dyes

Aromantic
www.aromantic.co.uk

Logona
www.logona.co.uk

Make your own

Neals Yard
Essential oils, vegetable and nut oils,
herbs, butters, and cream and shampoos
bases.
http://remedies.nealsyardremedies.com

Aromantic
One thousand ingredients, raw
materials, equipment, inspiration plus all
the information needed to make your
own natural, safe, cruelty-free cosmetics
and skin-care products.
www.aromantic.co.uk

Bay House Aromatics
Essential oils, vegetable oils, organically
certified oils, creams and shampoo
bases, bottles.
www.bay-house.co.uk

Cosmetics at Home
Information and materials for people
interested in hand-made natural
cosmetics and toiletries.
www.cosmeticsathome.co.uk

New Directions
Company selling pure essential oils,
certified organic oils, raw materials
(butters, clays, herbs, etc.) wholesale.
www.newdirectionsuk.com

Shopping Online

General stockists

Adilli
www.adili.com

Ecotopia
www.ecotopia.co.uk

Ecobtq
www.ecobtq.com

Ethical Superstore
www.ethicalsuperstore.com

Goodness Direct
www.goodnessdirect.co.uk
The Natural Store
www.thenaturalstore.co.uk

Bodycare and cosmetics

Beauty Naturals
www.beautynaturals.com

Pure Face Care
www.purefacecare.co.uk

Honesty Cosmetics
www.honestycosmetics.co.uk

There Must Be a Better Way
www.theremustbeabetterway.co.uk

Index